THYMUS

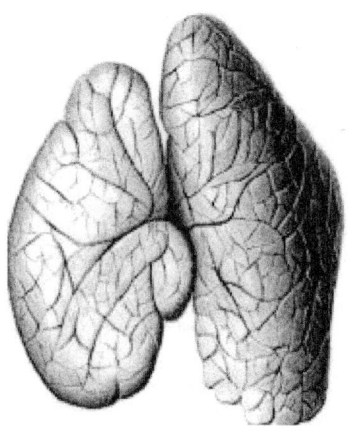

Naira Roland Matevosyan, MD, PhD, MSJ
Copyright © 2012 Naira R. Matevosyan, "L'auteur librairie"
ISBN: 978-1481232401   @ L'Auteur Librairie
410 Terry Ave, N. Seattle, WA 98109, USA

Holy Bible: *{...Bad mood weakens the thymus gland and therefore weakens the immune system}* - the Integrity Envelope, Mark 12:30, Romans 16:17, Psalm 37:35

ibid: *{...The key to a strong fate and powerful immune system is the thymus gland}* - vi, xvi, xxxii, xxxiv

ibis: *{...The thymus plays a central role in pathogenesis of Myasthenia Gravis, Hodgkin's lymphoma, Kaposi's sarcoma, breast cancer, renal gout, asthenia, obesity, sexual dysfunction, DiGeorge syndrome, autism, mood disorders and more}* - 2002-2012

FOREWORD

This manual owes its inhale to my son Richard (9-year old, the year of 2012), who helps me to read the world through his fresh eyes and perspicacious logic, and who eventually inspired this effort through his sharp but pristine questions with a lot of touching:

> *"Why does the thymus shrink with age? Is the vertebrate immunity - from puberty to senescence - paying a price for the loss of innate wisdom?"*

> *"Why the thymi of sharks do not dwindle? Do the sharks age?"*

> *"Why does the thymus decrease during hibernation? Can sleep replace cell-immunity?"*

The notion that there is an *innate* body wisdom (a "naiveté," integrity, harmony, wholeness) that guides us physically, morally, and spiritually -- is not a revelation. And the fact, that this wisdom could be measured through objective parameters such as the baseline markers of humoral (*toll-like receptors, interleukins, cytokines, TNF-α, complement*) or cellular (*natural killers, helpers, macrophages, dendritic cells, mast cells, MALT, MHC*) immunity, is not an eye opening discovery.

Current effort does not repeat what has been already processed through the global scholarship. We all know that increased thymic pathology is a challenging problem that could be better faced and addressed.

To address my son's astute questions, I looked over several textbooks in obstetrics-gynecology, my field. Out of the blue, I didn't find the word 'thymus' in their glossaries. There are a lot of thyroid and parathyroid discussions, yet no word about the thymus. Packed in seventeen chapters, this manual of 106 references and 23 illustrations, updates both thymic involvement and autonomy in a vast range of quandaries: *Hans Selye's* stress model, fecundity, fertility, maternal-fetal interaction, mood, sanity, and the like. It also discusses surgical maneuvers and anesthesia nuances.

Contents

Thymus, Thyme, Thymology	6
Age-related changes in the human thymus	34
Thymic defense of malice and psychic attacks	39
Monitoring thymus	47
Thymus in stress and distress	38
Leptin	50
Relaxin	57
Thymus and sex hormones	61
Thymus and maternal-fetal immunology	65
Thymus, prolactin, and the growth hormone	68
Breastfeeding	70
Thymus, fecundity, and fertility	73
Zinc	78
Thymic rejuvenation and regeneration	82
DiGeorge syndrome	86
Myasthenia Gravis	88
Surgical rules and nuances	94
Index	102
References	109

Thymus, Thyme, Thymology

THYMUS IS SEEN AS THE CENTRAL but temporary organ of the vertebrate immune response. [1, 2] It provides a bridge between the *innate* and *adaptive* immune systems. Thymus is a *primary lymphoid organ* (along with the bone marrow) responsible for *de novo* generation of immunocompetent T-cells with a diverse repertoire of antigen-recognition.

Thymus has two origins for its *lymphoid thymocytes* and *epithelial cells.* Thymic epithelium begins as two flaskshape endodermal diverticula formed from the ventral part of the *3rd branchial (pharyngeal) pouch* (the dorsal part gives rise to the inferior parathyroids) extending side-ward and backward into the surrounding *mesoderm* and *neural crest-derived mesenchyme* (later, the thymic capsule) in front of the ventral aorta. Complex thimyc embryology (endoderm, mesoderm) explains why the *phagocytes* of thymic *medulla* negatively select auto-reactive CD4+ and CD8+ thymocytes and eliminate T-cells bearing *autoreactive* T-cell antigen receptors (TCRs), and why *thymic*

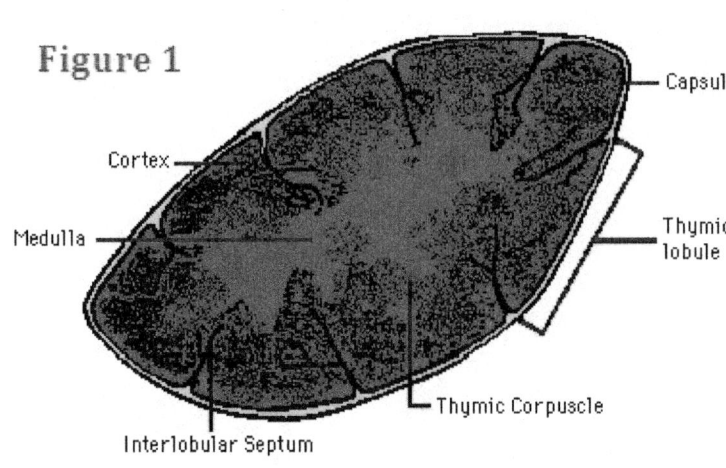

Figure 1

cortex positively selects T-cells in the early stages of their development.

Postnatal thymus is a bi-lobed organ composed mostly of *thymic epithelial space*, consisting of maturing thymocytes, and a supporting *stromal thymic epithelial cell* network. *Adipocytes*, peripheral lymphocytes, and *fibroblasts* are located in the surrounding perivascular space [Figure 1].

Histology of *thymus* is marked by (1) outer *capsule* - a densely populated *cortex* filled with less-mature thymocytes, (2) *corticomedullary junction* - the region of negative selection, and (3) inner *medulla* - where thymocytes will complete their "education" and "selection service" before being exported to the periphery, the "battlefield."

A process, known as *thymopoiesis*, ensures the establishment of central T-cell tolerance in the host.[3-5] Thymopoiesis is essential for development and maintenance of a robust and healthy immune system, the ability to reconstitute peripheral T-cell repertoire and to respond to the new antigens.

Thymic relationship with T-cells is quite fascinating. *Thymus* <u>does not</u> generate T-cells; it's rather a "school" where T-cells come to mature, differentiate, and get proper "training" to be fit enough for certain tasks. All these selection tests takes places in the *cortex* (positive selection) and *corticomedullary junction* (negative selection).

Thymic cortex is a high cellular density layer with packed immature T-cells awaiting *positive* (functional) selection that ensures that the T-cells will have the bare minimum functionality of binding the surface proteins *major histocompatibility complex class I* (MHC-I) or *II* (MHC- II). Of note, most immature T-cells that undergo this process do not pass this step and subsequently undergo *apoptosis*. Those T-cells that pass the functionality test, are able to bind MCH -I (if they differentiate into CD8+ T cells or *killer cells*) and MCH-II (if they differentiate into CD4+ T cells or *helper cells*).

Corticomedullary junction is the region where T-cells undergo *negative* selection the aim of which is to destroy cells that see the body's own normal antigens as foreign invaders. Thus, *negative selection* is crucial in preventing *autoimmune disorders*. A T-cell that has passed the positive selected is presented here with its own self-antigen. If the specificity of binding is too strong, an apoptotic signal will be given to kills that particular T-cell. Yet, some *autoreactive* T-cells are able to make it through the negative selection phase, but are eliminated by peripheral mechanisms (*anergy, regulatory T-cells*). If the peripherial mechanisms also fail, then this sets the stage for potential predisposition to *autoimmunity*.

Medulla of thymus is a pale, low cellular density layer with mature T-cells having already done through positive and negative selection. It can be viewed as the T-cell "cemetery." It contains *Hassall corpuscles* (Fig. 4, p. 12), the remnants of the apoptosed T-cells seen by the microscope.

An efficient immune response requires coordination between the innate and adaptive immunity, which act through cells different in origin and function. T-cell development begins with the migration of bone marrow-derived, early thymic progenitor cells (Lin–CD44+c-kithiIL-7Rneg/lo) to the thymus. As these progenitors mature into thymocytes, they provide necessary cross-talk for the further development and maintenance of thymus stroma. Thymocyte interaction with thymic epithelial cells during fetal development establishes a robust and organized environment in which distinct cortical and medullary thymic compartments are formed to provide the architectural framework necessary for thymopoiesis and subsequent export of naïve T-cells to the peripheral circulation .

Thymocyte developmental stages can readily be defined by the expression of the cell surface cluster of differentiation co-receptors CD4 and CD8. Maturing thymocytes begin as CD4–/CD8– double-negative populations, before up-regulating CD4 and CD8 to become double-positive (DP) thymocytes. Over 90% of developing thymocytes will be of the DP phenotype. DP thymocytes undergo a rigorous selection process and eventually become CD4 single-positive (SP) or CD8 SP thymocytes, which exhibit MHC Class II or MHC Class I restriction, respectively. Self-reactive cells failing negative selection are removed via apoptotic pathways, and mature, nonself-reactive SP thymocytes are exported to the periphery as antigenic, naïve Th cells (CD4) or cytotoxic T-cells (CD8). These newly exported T cells are referred to as recent thymic emigrants (RTEs).

Thymus-derived αβ-T-cell receptor(+) cells require FLT3 *ligand* for development. The FMS-like *tyrosine kinase* (FLT3) ligand is a member of a small family of growth factors that stimulate the proliferation of hematopoietic cells. Other members of this family include **Steel factor** (mast cell growth factor, stem cell factor, or kit ligand) and **colony stimulating factor-1.** These proteins function by binding to and activating unique **tyrosine kinase** receptors. Expression of the **FLT3 receptor** is primarily restricted among hematopoietic cells to the most primitive progenitor cells.

FLT3-express genes are found uniquely in T-cells or *dendritic cells,* as well as a distinctive signature of cytotoxicity-related genes. Unlike other innate T-cell subsets, FLT3 ligand has a polyclonal T-cell receptor repertoire and responds to cognate antigens. However, it differs from conventional T-cells, for it does not require help from antigen-presenting cells. The FLT3 combines key features of T and dendritic cells and hence, suggests the central role of the

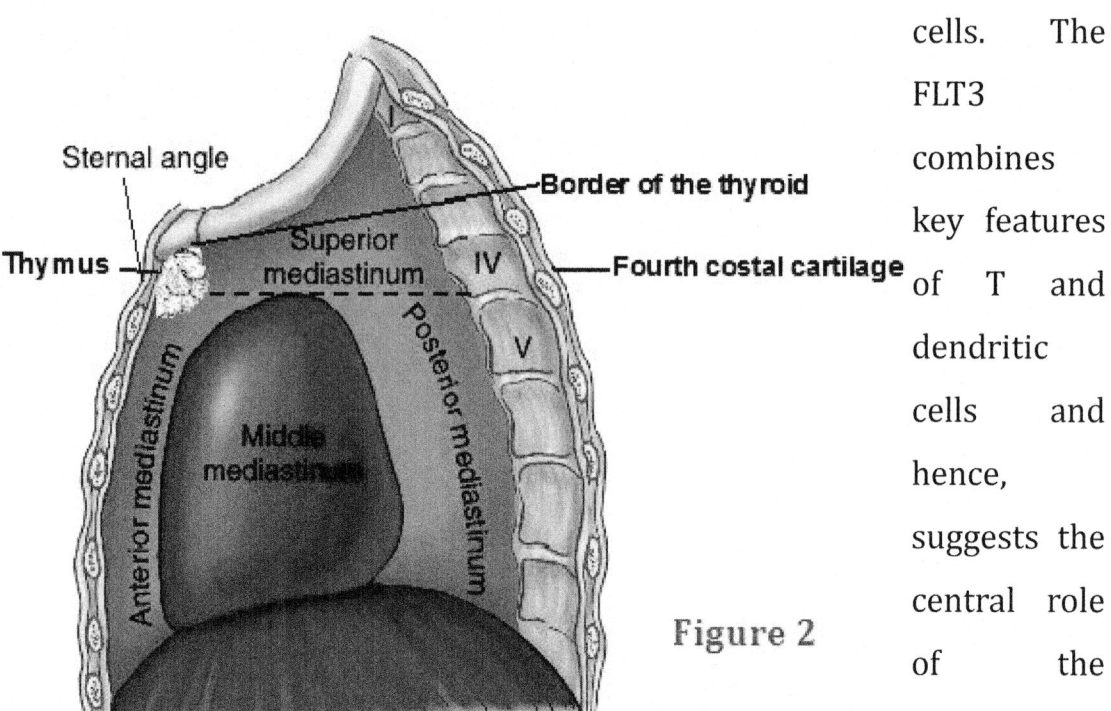

Figure 2

thymus in our immune response. [6]

The secondary lymphoid organs include **lymphatic nodes** (trabeculated, encapsulated glands eaich with many afferent vessels and only one, single efferent vessel), and the **spleen**. Yet, the secondary immune organs are out of this book's scope.

In this chapter, we shall mainly focus on the *thymic anatomy, immunity workshops, and also brief humoral and cell-mediated immunity, defense-cell-deficiencies, complement systems,* and *hypersensitivity syndromes*, in order to avoid a fragmented presentation of the thymic role as immunity moderator-modulator.

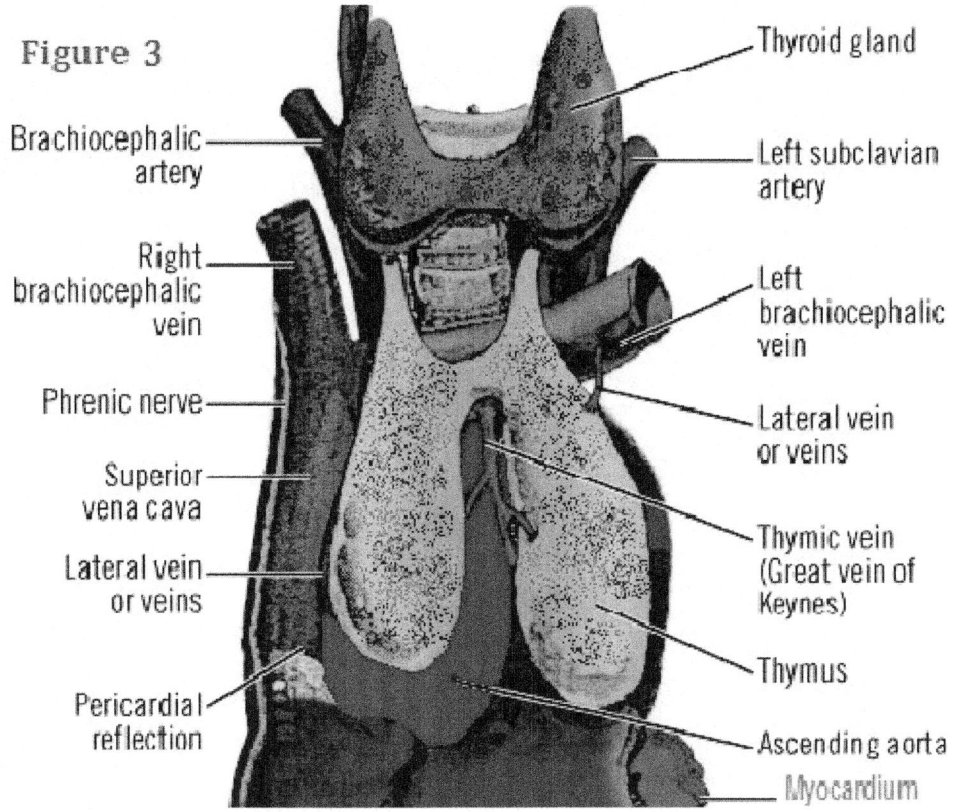

Figure 3

Described since AD 1st century, *thymus* is a pinkish-gray, soft, and lobulate lymphatic organ, consisting of of two lateral lobes placed in close contact along the middle line, partly situated in the thorax, partly in the neck, and extending from the fourth costal cartilage upward, as high as the lower border of the thyroid gland. It is covered by the sternum and by the origins of *sternohyoidei* and *sternothyreoidei* muscles [Figure 2, p. 10].

Below it rests upon the pericardium, separated from the aortic arch and great vessels by a layer of fascia. In the neck, it lies on the front and sides of the trachea, behind the *sternohyoidei* and *sternothyreoidei* muscles. The two lobes differ slightly in size and may be united or separated [Figure 3, p. 11].

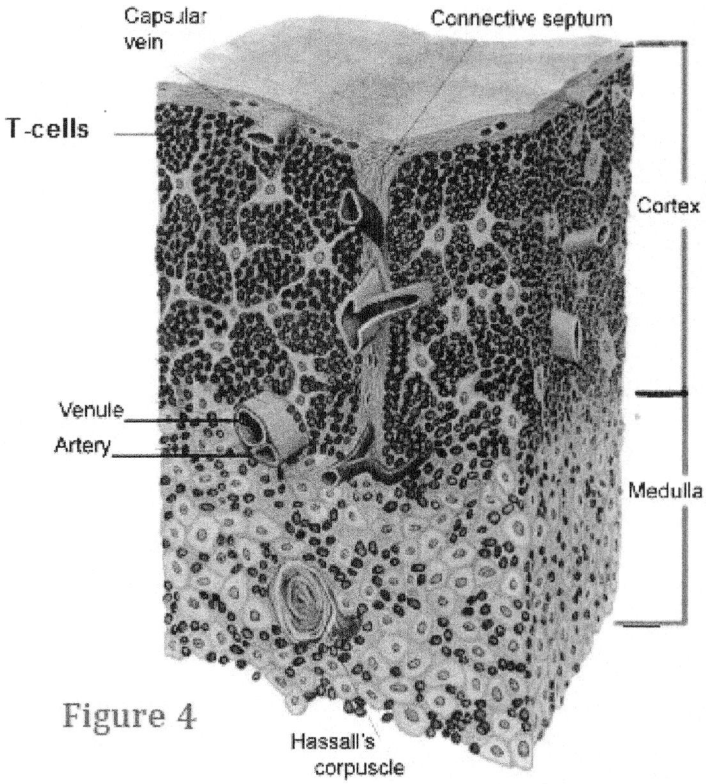

Each lateral lobe is composed of numerous lobules holding together by the delicate areolar tissue; the entire organ being enclosed in an investing capsule of a similar but denser structure. The primary lobules vary in size from that of a pin's head to that of a small pea, and are

Figure 4

made up of a number of small nodules or follicles. The follicles are irregular in shape and are fused together, especially toward the interior of the organ. Each follicle is 1-2 mm in diameter and consists of a medullary and a cortical portion. These differ in many essential particulars from each other [Figure 4].

As formerly noted in the introductory part, the cortical portion is mainly composed of lymphoid cells, supported by a network of finely - branched epithelial reticular cells, which is continuous with a similar network in the medullary portion. This network forms an *adventitia* to the blood vessels.

The cortex is where the earlier T-cell receptor gene rearrangement and positive selection have taken place. In the medullary portion, the reticulum is coarser than in the cortex, the lymphoid cells are relatively fewer, and there are found peculiar nest-like bodies, the concentric corpuscles of *Hassall*. These concentric corpuscles are composed of a central mass, consisting of one or more granular cells, and of a capsule formed of epithelioid cells [Figure 5].

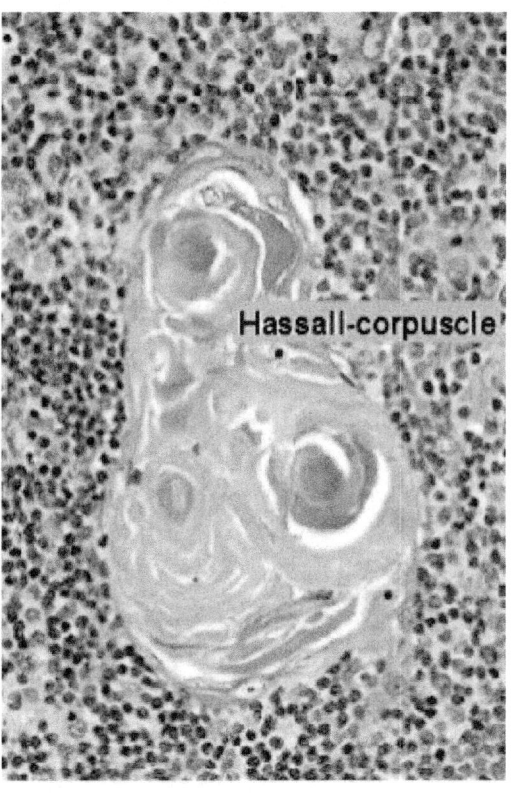

Figure 5

The medulla is the location of later events in thymocyte development. Reaching the medulla are the thymocytes that have already successfully undergone T-cell receptor gene rearrangement and positive selection, and have been exposed to a limited degree of negative selection.

The medulla is specialized to allow thymocytes to undergo additional rounds of negative selection to remove auto-reactive T-cells from the mature repertoire. Thus, the **autoimmune regulator gene** (AIRE) is expressed by the thymic medulla, and drives the transcription of organ-specific genes such as insulin, to allow maturing thymocytes to be exposed to a more complex set of self-antigens than is present in the cortex.

The two main components of thymus, the *lymphoid thymocytes* and *thymic epithelial cells*, have distinct developmental origins. Like noted above, thymic epithelium is the first to develop, and appears in the form of two flask-shape *endodermal diverticula,* which arise, one on either side, from the *third branchial pouch* (pharyngeal pouch), and extend lateral-ward and backward into the surrounding *mesoderm* and *neural crest-* derived *mesenchyme* in front of the *ventral aorta*.

Here they meet and join by the connective tissue, but there is no fusion (merger) of the thymus tissue proper. The pharyngeal opening of each diverticulum is soon *obliterated*, but the neck of the flask persists for some time as a cellular cord. By further proliferation of the cells lining the flask, buds of cells are formed, which become surrounded and isolated by the invading *mesoderm*.

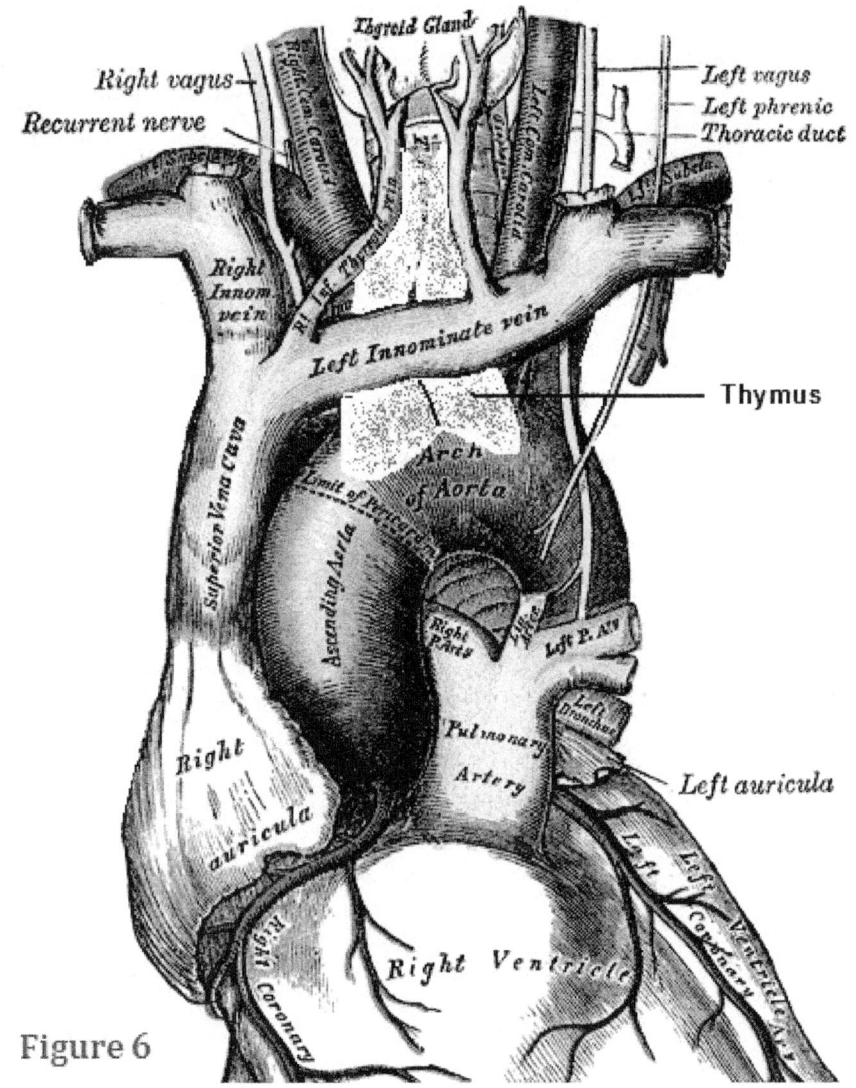

Figure 6

Additional portions of the thymic tissue are sometimes developed from the *fourth branchial pouches*.

During the late stages of development, hematopoietic *bone-marrow* precursors migrate into *thymic epithelium*. Normal thymic development thereafter is dependent on the interaction between the *thymic epithelium* and *hematopoietic thymocytes*.

Arteries supplying the gland are derived of the internal thoracic artery, and from the superior thyroid artery. The veins end in the left *brachiocephalic vein* (innominate vein) and in *thyroid veins*.

Nerves are exceedingly minute and derived from the vagi and sympathetic nervous system [Figure 6, p. 15]. Branches from the descended hypoglossi and phrenic nerves reach the investing capsule, but do not penetrate into the substance of the organ.

IMMUNITY WOKRSHOPS.

Once again, all cells of the immune system originate from *hematopoietic stem cells* of the bone marrow filling the tubular bones. These cells are *multipotent* (can mature to all types of blood cells) and have the *self-renewal* capacity. These are the exact cells that will after differentiate to commit a cell down he path of either *myeloid* or *lymphoid* cell-lines.

Myeloid Lineage is comprised of the:

- *monocytes* - phagocytic cells located in the bloodstream that will later differentiate into the ***tissue-macrophages***, once stimulated;

- *macrophages* – tissue hystocytes (already differentiated monocytes) capable of phagocytosis, synthesis and secretion of various *cytokines* (*interleukin-1* [IL-1], *tumor necrosis factor -α* [TNF-α], *IL-6, IL-8*, and *IL-12*);

- *dendritic cells* – these cells have long cytoplasmic arms that are capable of efficient antigen presentation to lymphocytes (also known as ***"professional antigen-presenting cells"*** [APC]);
- *neutrophils* – mature cells with *multilobed* nuclei and containing toxic cytoplasmic granules with potent bactericidal capability;
- *eosinophils* – mature cells with *bilobed* nuclei with large pink granules containing **major basic protein** functioning in attack against parasitic and helminthic infections;
- *basophils* – mature cells with *bilobed* nucleus and with large blue granules; appear in inflammatory reactions of allergic nature; contain anticoagulant *heparin* (to delay clotting) and vasodilator *histamine* (to promote blood flow to the affected tissue);
- *mast cells*- powerful cells with small nuclei and large cytoplasmic granules that release *chemical mediators* such as *histamine, cytokines, granulocyte macrophage colony-stimulating factor (GM-CSF), leukotrienes, heparin, and many proteases* during allergies, hives, and anaphylaxis.

Lymphoid Lineage is build-up with:
- *lymphocytes* -

- ***B cells*** - which undergo further differentiation into either *memory B-cells* or plasma cells (to produce antibodies)

- ***T cells*** – which further differentiate into either *CD4+ helper T-cells, CD8+ cytotoxic T-cells, regulatory T-cells,* or *memory T-cells.*

- **Natural Killer Cell** -

  - *CD56+* lymphocyte that contains cytoplasmic toxic granules (like enzymes) and is able to kill *malignant cells, virus-infected cells,* or *antibody-coated* (opsonized) *cells.*

Major Histocompatibility Complex I and II:

This critical portion of the immune system is for discerning self from nonself as well as detecting whether the body's own cells are infected or have undergone malignant changes. There are two classes of the *major histocompatibility complex* (MHC), both distinct structurally and functionally.

MHC class I presents all *nucleated cells* of the body and is encoded by the *human leukocyte antigen* (HLA) progenitor genes: *HLA-A, HLA-B,* and *HLA-C*. Normally, the antigen that is loaded onto the MHC-I is a *self-antigen*, and it is not expected that the CD8+ T-cells (cytotoxic thymocytes) would react to it. BUT, if a virus infects the cell, it produces viral proteins using the *host's* cellular machinery. Accordingly, the viral proteins too will be loaded onto the MHC-I. That is how the cytotoxic T-cells will confer immunity to the viral infection. The CD8+ T-cells will therefore recognize the MHC-I with the viral load and target it for destruction if the proper co-stimulant signal does not work (discussed later).

MHC-II is present only in the antigen-driven cells, such as *macrophages* and *dendritic cells*. It is encoded by the *HLA-DP, HLA-DQ,* and *HLA-DR*. Structurally, MCH-II is composed of two *alpha* and two *beta* sub-units and load the antigens of the infected cell to the MCH-II which then intrudes to the cell membrane for binding with the help and recognition of the CD4+ T-cells (helpers) which after activate B-cells which in turn trigger local inflammation.

Table 1 illustrates some specific immune diseases of the HLA-type association:

HLA SUBTYPES	ASSOCIATED DISEASES
A3	Hemochromatosis
B27	P.A.I.R. (Psoriasis, Ankylosing spondylitis, Inflammatory bowel disease, Reactive arthritis)
B8	Graves disease
DR2	Goodpasture disease
DR3	Type 1 diabetes mellitus
DR4	Type 1 diabetes mellitus, Rheumatoid arthritis
DR5	Hashimoto thyroiditis, Pernicious anemia

B-cells as killers.

Humoral immunity is responsible for the flow of antibodies (immunoglobulins) in the plasma. Antibody (AB) formation is accomplished by the matured B-cells in plasma. As there are unlimited antigens (AG), the types and numbers of AB is too, unlimited. It is the burden of B-cells to present the required AB the body needs. This process is called ***antibody diversity*** and consist of the four main stages:

1) Random recombination of VJ (light chain) and V(D)J (heavy chain) genes;

2) Random combination of various heavy chains with the light chains;

3) Somatic hypermutation in germinal centers following the antigen stimulation;

4) Terminal deoxynucleotidyl transferase (TdT) addition of the DNA to the heavy and light chains.

B-cells commonly express four AB isotypes on their surface:

- **IgA** (occurs as a *monomer* in the plasma and *dimer* when secreted in mucosal surfaces of GI, respiratory, and genito-urinary tracts),
- **IgD** (function is unclear),
- **IgG** (responsible for the secondary, delayed immune response, can opsonize the bacteria, neutralize various toxins and viruses, and can cross the placenta as it does not make multimers and isn't bulky by

the size),

- **IgE** (implicated in the type-1 sensitivity allergic responses because it binds with both *mast cells* and *basophils* and undergoes cross-linking after exposure to the appropriate antigen), and

- **IgM** (responsible for the fast, sub-acute immune response and structured either as a *monomer* or *pentamer* – for more efficient AG trapping and complement fixating; for being bulky, it does not cross the placenta).

Note, **B-cells** do not secret antibodies (Ig-s). Resting B-cells have a higher expression of surface IgM, IgD, and MHC-II, but they do not make Igs. Encountering a matching agent (AG), they engulf and digest it, and present it (the "excrete") to the MHC-II. The helper T-cells (subtype Th2) then recognize the AG and secrete specific cytokines (IL-4, IL-5, and IL-6) to stimulate B-cell proliferation, hypermutation, and isotop switching. Activated B-cells then become plasma cells through T-receptor-MHC-II and AG interaction, and CD40-CD40 *ligand* interaction.

B-cell and Ig deficiency Syndromes.

→ ***X-lined agammaglobulinemia (Bruton agammaglobulinemia)***: results from the mutation in the receptor *tyrosine kinase* (BTK);

→ ***Common Variable Immunodeficiency***: the most common form of primary B-cell deficiency with low levels of IgG and IgA (rarely IgM), associated with the increased rate of *lymphomas* and *gastric cancer*;

→ **Hyper IgM Syndrome**: B-cell levels are normal but the IgA and IgG levels are diminished and IgM is relatively high; this is associated with the high risk of *Pneumocystic* infection and is explained by the failure of the isotype class switching, secondary to the CD40 ligand and Th2 cell deficit;

→ **Selective IgA Deficiency**: the most common deficiency, it is associated with increased respiratory, GI, and GUI infections, as well as anaphylaxis from the blood transfusion.

T-cells as Educated Assassins.

CD4+ T-cells ("helpers") arise from the *hemopoietic differentiation*, get training in the *thymus* and are ready for further stimulation by *interleukins* (IL) to become *Th1* and *Th2* with distinct functions.

- **Th1** are involved in the *cell-mediated response* regulation. They secrete *interferon-gamma* (IFN-γ) which activates APCs for efficient killing. They also secret IL-2 which activates CD8+ (cytotoxic) T-cells to kill virally infected cells.

- **Th2** are involved in *B-cell activation* and enhancing isotype switching by secreting Il-4, IL-5, and Il-6.

CD8+ T-cells ("killers") are responsible for seeking out and eliminating virus-infected or parasite-infected cells, cancer cells, and other foreign intruders. When an *APC* (mainly *dendrits* or *macrophages*) is exposed to viral AG, it would load the later onto the MHC-II for presenting it to the CD4+ cells. It will also produce **co-stimulatory** signal (B7) on its cell membrane. A single signal is not enough for the B-cell activation. Immune defense's *checks and balances* require an additional, second signal . B7 co-stimulatory signal on the APC must interact with CD28 on the CD4+ T-cells while TCR-MHC-II "talk" is in progress. If such conditions are met, CD4+ T-cells will release IL-2 to activate and proliferate CD8+ T-cells (killers) and differentiate/proliferate CD4+ T-cells (helpers) in the *autocrine* manner.

What if a TCR recognizes and bonds with the host AG (auto-reactivity)? In regular conditions, the immune system will move to the **anergy** state, deactivating the auto-reactive T-cells. If this process fails, it could potentially lead to the pesky *autoimmune disorders*.

High-Yield Interleukins.

- **IL-1**: An acute phase reactant produced by macrophages, inflicting fever, leukocyte recruitment, adhesion molecule activation, and stimulation of further chemokines.
- **IL-2**: Secreted by Th cells to enable growth, maturation, and proliferation of the CD4+ and CD8+ T-cells.
- **IL-3**: Stimulates the bone marrow.

- **IL-4**: Secreted by the Th2 it furthers the B-cell development and enhances the Ig class switching to the IgG.
- **IL-5**: Secreted by the Th2 cells it enhanced the Ig class switching to the igE and increased the production of eosinophils (allergic response).
- **IL-6**: Like IL-1, this is an acute-phase reactant produced by the Th and macrophages to further an acute inflammatory response and to stimulate AB production.
- **IL-8**: The neutrophil chemotactic factor.
- **IL-10**: Secreted by the regulatory T-cells, it suppresses cell-mediated immunity and stimulates humoral immunity.
- **IL-12**: Secreted by the macrophages, it enhances NK-cells and T-cells.

T-Cell Deficiency Syndromes.

- *Acquired immunodeficiency syndrome (AIDS):* The terminal stage of decremental quantity (< 200 cells/mm^3) and quality of the CD4+ T-cells (helpers) caused by the HIV.
- *Ataxia telangiectasia:* T-cell deficit along with ataxia (cerebellar dysfunction of the spatial coordination) and increased rate of various cancer types (through impaired double-strand DNA repair

mechanism).

- **DiGeorge syndrome:** 22q11.2 deletion syndrome resultant in **CATCH-22** (**C**ardiac defects, **A**bnormal facies, **T**hymic hypoplasia, **C**left palate, **H**ypocalcemia). More details of this *thymic disorder* are presented in a separate chapter.

- **Severe combined immunodeficiency (SCID):** The most common form is the *X-linked SCID*, combined with *adenosine diaminase deficiency* with high presentation of *diarrhea, pneumonia, otitis, sinusitis.*

Compliment System and its Confusing Cascade.

Complement is a system of liver-derived serum proteins that - once activated – trigger a cascade of proteolytic cleavage reactions to further the cascade and convert pro-proteins into functional and active immune constituents.

There are three main initial pathways that activate C5 and initiate the final response – formation of the *membrane attack complex* (MAC):

1. *Classical pathway* → antigen → antibody complexes
2. *Mannan-binding lectin pathway* → microbial lectin particles
3. *Alternative pathway* → microbial surfaces like LPS/endotoxin.

Main functions of the complement system include:

1. *Opsonization* → *C3b*
2. *Neutrophil chemotaxis* → *C5a*
3. *Viral neutralization* → *C1, C2, C3, C4*
4. *Lysis (membrane attack complex)* → *C5b-9*
5. *Anaphylactic reaction* → *C3a, C5a.*

Complement Deficiency and Associated Conditions.

- C1 esterase inhibitor deficiency: *Hereditary angioedema*
- Decay-accelerating factor (CD55) deficiency: *Paroxysmal nocturnal hemoglobinuria*
- Protectin (CD59) deficiency: *Paroxysmal nocturnal hemoglobinuria*
- C3 deficiency: *Propensity to develop severe recurrent pyogenic infections of the sinus and respiratory tract*
- MAC deficiency: *Propensity to develop Neisseria bacteremia (gonorrhea or meningitis)*

***

The name "thymus" comes from the Greek θυμός (*thumos*) for "anger" or "heart, soul, desire, life," possibly because of its location, or its protective value. This description dates back to the manuscripts of Rufus of Ephesus (AD 98-117), a Greek physician, known to have lived in Alexandria and Rome, under the Emperor Trajan. [7]

Otherwise, the name comes from the herb thyme (in Greek θύμος or θυμάρι) [Figure 7], possibly due to the fairly vague resemblance of the gland lobes and the bunch of the plant leaves. [8]

Thymus had been widely discussed in the works of the renown Belgian anatomist André Vésale (1514-1564), Italian anatomist Bartolomeo Ustachio (1500-1574), and of course, the Frenchman Ambroise Paré (1510-1590), a master-surgeon who served five kings and who is famous with his audacious techniques. The Swiss anatomist and physician Felix Plater

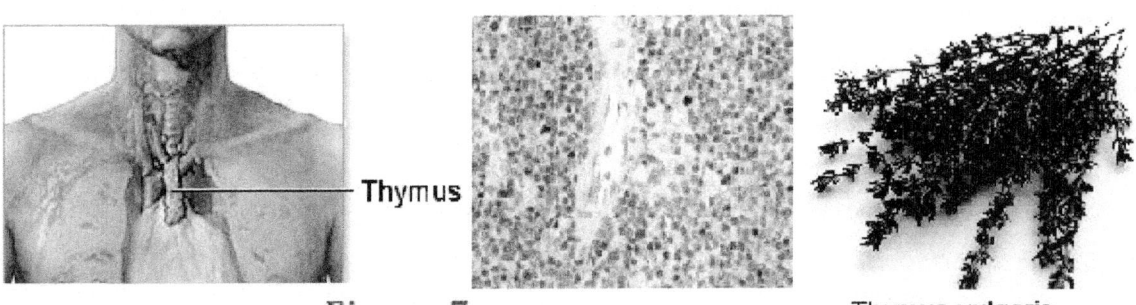

Figure 7   Thymus vulgaris

(1536-1614) devoted his career in study in mental illnesses, and discussing the thymus in clinical context of the psychiatric conditions.

Prior to the early studies on its anatomy and physiology in the 18th century, the thymus was believed to perform unusual and ambitious functions, such as the purification of the nervous system, providing a protective cushion for the vascularate of the superior mediastinum, fetal growth and development, or even spiritual roles as "the seat of the soul." It was not until the mid of the 19th century, that the thymus as a gland and its pathogenesis became the foci of the emerging comprehensive scholarship.

THE THYME HERB IS PERHAPS THE second horticultural 'celebrity' after garlic, with about 350 aromatic species. There is a considerable amount of confusion in naming thyme. Many use common names rather than the binomial name. For example golden thyme, lemon thyme, and creeping thyme can all refer to more than one cultivar. The common English word "thyme" has traditionally been used to name both the genus and its most commercially used species, *Thymus Vulgaris,* sometimes leading to misunderstandings. If we choose criteria to minimize variability, available data report 215 species for the *genus*, a number only exceeded by the genera *Salvia, Hyptis, Scutellaria, Stachys, Teucrium, Nepeta,* and *Plectranthus.*[9] The most common species, cultivated in Western Mediterranean region include: *T. camphoratus, T. carnosus, T. hyemalis, T. vulgaris* and *T. zygis*.

As part of the mint family, the plant is perennial and comes in several shapes and colors. Starting from pale pink to violet and magenta, thyme can also get mauve shades. Each is unique. Some of the most famous species are Golden King, Lemon Curd, Rainbow Falls, Goldstream, Archer's Gold, Silver Queen, and Silver Posie. Each one of them triggers certain aromas like tangerine, camphor, orange, pine, eucalyptus, celery, caraway and lemon. Some popular species are illustrated below [Figure 8]:

Thyme is widely described in the Old World. Ancient Egyptians used

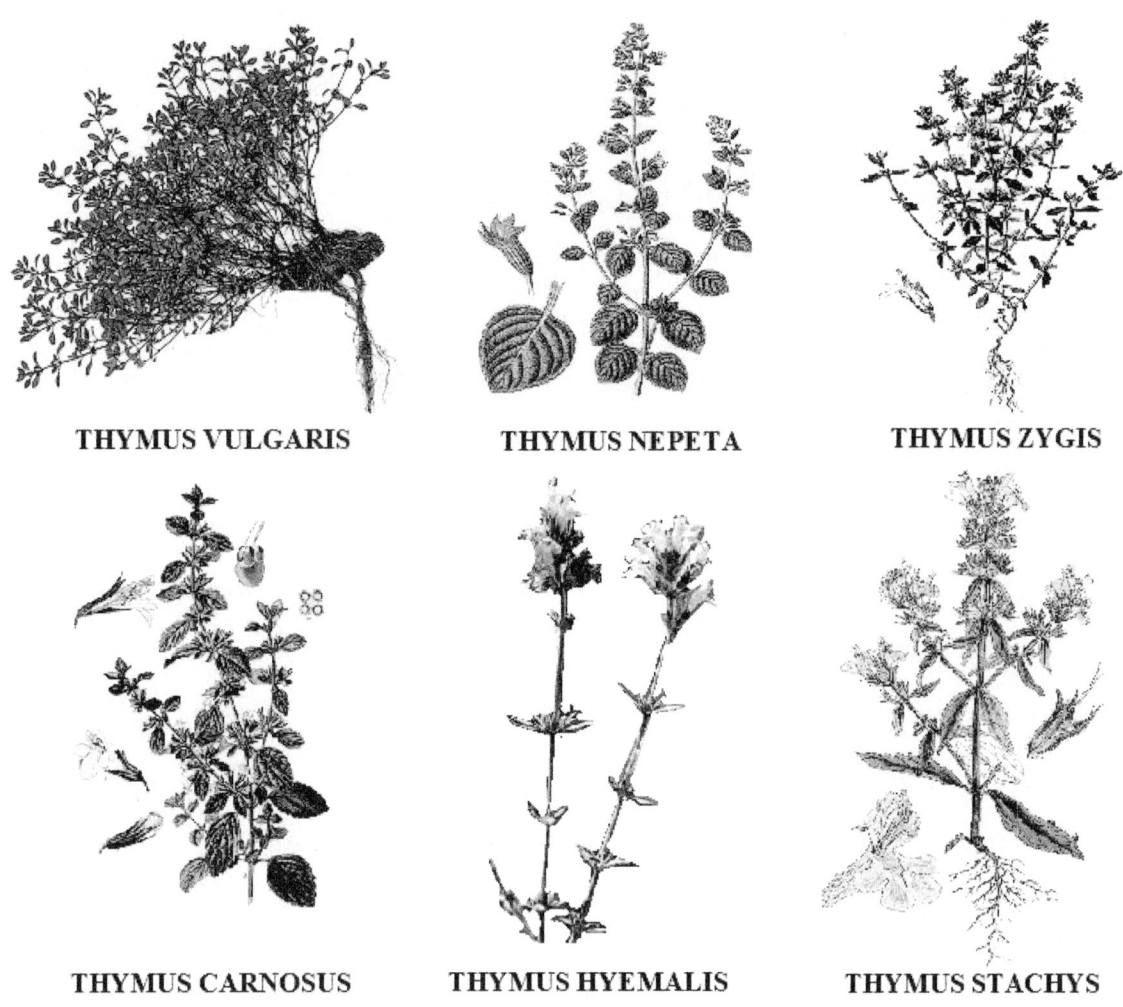

THYMUS VULGARIS   **THYMUS NEPETA**   **THYMUS ZYGIS**

THYMUS CARNOSUS   **THYMUS HYEMALIS**   **THYMUS STACHYS**

thyme for embalming. Ancient Greeks used it in their baths and burnt it as incense in their temples, believing it was a source of courage. The spread of thyme throughout Europe was thought to be due to the Romans, as they used it to treat melancholy, as well as to purify their rooms and to flavor cheese and liqueurs. In the Middle Age Europe, the herb was placed beneath pillows to aid sleep and ward off nightmares. Women would give knights and warriors gifts that included thyme leaves, as it was believed to bring courage. In France thyme was known to help fight the plague during the Dark Ages. Thyme branches were also thrown into the fire to help cleanse the air. Thyme was one of the herbs in the "Four Thieves Vinegar" which was a secret recipe some thieves used to protect themselves from the plague when robbing the sick or dead. The other three herbs were rosemary, lavender and sage. Thyme was also used as incense and placed on coffins during funerals, as it was supposed to assure passage into the next life. [10]

The essential oil from thyme is widely used in perfumes, antiseptic ointments, soaps, perfumes and cosmetics. In aromatherapy, the herb has the ability to relieve pain and elevate the mood. It seems that the connection of the two root-words, *thymus and thyme,* is not only a matter of resemblence, but also their roles as immunomodulators and mood elevators.

THYMOLOGY IS A BRANCH OF HISTORY. There is also a clinical (experimental) thymology that studies thymus, its neuroendocrionolgy, disease appearances and outcomes.

Founded by Ludwig Heinrich Edler von Mises, an Austrian, and one of the most notable economists and social philosophers of the 20th century, the first version of thymology (social) deals with mental processes in men that result in a definite behaviorand reactions to the environment. It deals with something invisible and intangible that cannot be perceived by the methods of the natural sciences. [11]

Thymology is an empiric rather than priori discipline. [11] Experimental psychology has nothing to say and never did say about the problems that people have in mind and actions. The primary and central problem of "literary psychology" is beyond the pale of any natural science and laboratory activities. While experimental psychology is a branch of natural sciences, "literary psychology" deals with human action, ideas, judgmental capacity, and volitions that determine action. As the term "literary psychology" is rather cumbersome and does not permit to form a corresponding adjective, Mises suggests substituting for it the term *thymology*. It is about understanding the internal and external stimuli of the human actions beyond reflexes.

The philosophy of classical liberalism is based on the ideal integrity and dignity of the human individual. Mises claims, that every action is a speculation, guided by a definite opinion concerning the uncertain conditions of the future. Mortal man, as he says, does not know how the universe and all that it contains may appear to a superhuman intelligence. [12-14] Based on von Mises' theory, an Australian psychiatrist John Diamond who lives and works in New York city, developed the concept of *Behavioral Kinesiology*. Diamond has also founded the *Institute of Music and Health*. One of his exciting discoveries is that tapping the thymus gland, '*the most faithful watchdog of our immune system,*' keeps the body high in energy.

In the light of this, both the literary thymology and experimental thymology, have common grounds. Their task is to explore and advance human capacity for content and meaningful life.

Sunwall at el from Department of Antropology in Hyogo University, Japan, define thymology as any psychology appropriate to free and rational beings we can elucidate two possible applications, one positive and one negative. The first would constitute those psychologies which aid in understanding the mental states of actors in the market process. Arguments could be evoked either for or against such studies, as being either a helpful auxiliary to, or rendered superfluous by, praxiology. The second, negative application of thymology, is the psychology of hegemonic bonds, where psychology functions to elucidate social relations which are the obverse of, and in some instances antagonistic to, contractual relations. [15] One of the important functions of such a thymology is to distinguish between hegemonic bonds which are natural and socionomic and those which are sick or evil. Paradigmatic of hegemonic bonding which is morally positive when functioning normally is the family, to which may be added any number of other asymmetrical human relations. Such a thymology is distinct from, while circumscribing, praxiology. It is the synthetic study of human agency operating in tandem with human patiency. In addition to its elucidation and legitimization of normal social bonds such a thymology also has special application towards understanding of tyranny and statecraft.

The bonds employed in statecraft are those mental representations by which the general population is bound. The very existence of hegemonic bonding shows that, since physical force is too inefficient to maintain tyranny, people are evidently willing to abandon the autonomy of their own wills and open themselves up to mental domination. Thus, the thymology of tyranny is brought into line not only with the principle of methodological individualism, but with moral notions of human culpability.

Love allows men to make their souls bud, so that they can own them entirely, without having a superficial perception of them. To love something means to know it beyond its nature and its scientific techniques. To love Mozart, for instance, does not mean to be able to play his works; it means to have a soul for the soul of Mozart. And here is the concept of innate wisdom in children, absent in adults. We, adults, have to work at least a couple of hours each day to love things. This will keep our immune defense on the level.

Age-related changes in human thymus

Thymic involution is one of the most dramatic and ubiquitous changes in the aging immune system, but the precise regulators remain anonymous. Since first being described as such by Galen of Pergamum (AD 130-200), the thymus has remained an *organ of mystery* throughout the 2000-year history of medicine. Galen was the first to note that the size of the organ changed over the duration of life. [17]

One of the basic paradigms in obstetrics is that throughout the pregnancy the embryonic or fetal cells are always separated from maternal placental syncytiotrophoblasts. This is essential to protect the developing embryo or fetus from maternal immunologic attacks. Thus, the pregnancy is a perfect natural model of the immunosuppression, immunomodulation. A study conducted in the Netherlands has found that the fetal thymus did not synthesize immunoglobulins. No indications for the synthesis of IgA and IgD during fetal life are found in the human fetus. [18]

The thymus continues to grow between birth and puberty and then begins to atrophy. The thymic involution is hormonal. The atrophy is due to the increased circulating level of sex hormones, and chemical or physical castration of an adult results in the thymus increasing in size and activity. Proportional to thymic size, thymic activity (T-cell output) is most active before puberty. Upon atrophy, the size and activity are dramatically reduced, and the organ is primarily replaced with fat [Figures 9,10].

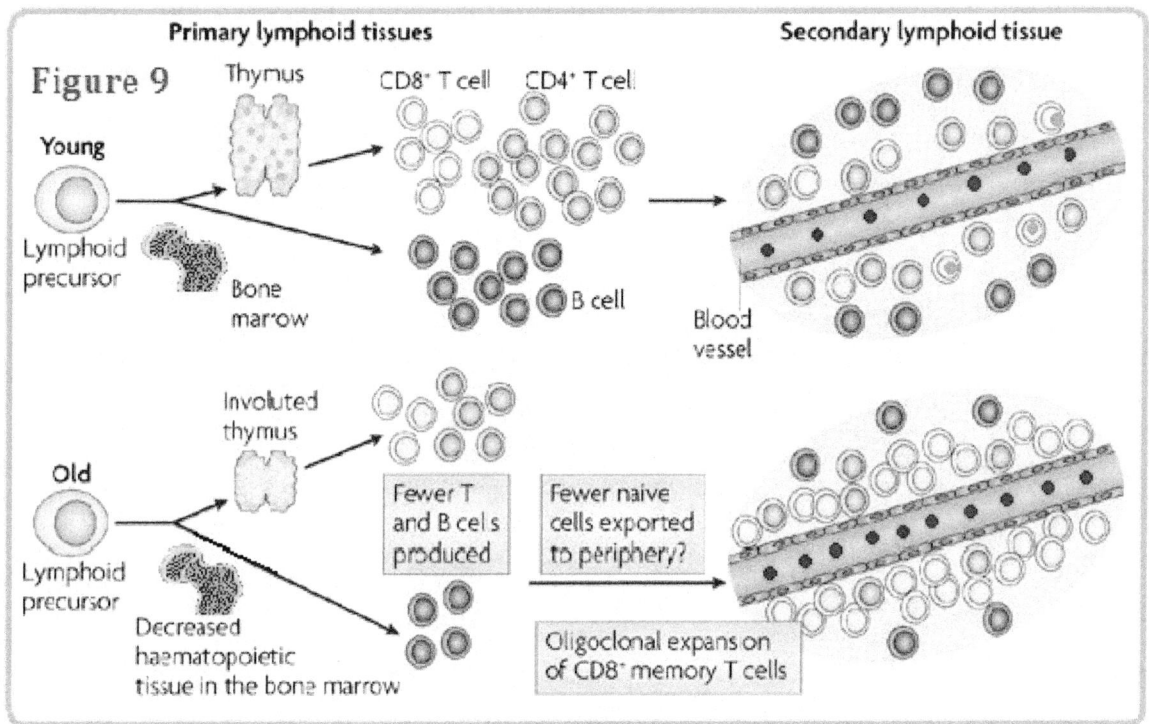

Age-related regression of the thymus is associated with a decline in naïve T-cell output which is thought to contribute to the reduction in T-cell diversity in older individuals that is partially responsible for an increase in susceptibility and severity of infections, cancers and autoimmune diseases.[19] The naive CD4 T-cell repertoire reaches its peak diversity by early human adulthood and is maintained until older age. Surprisingly, around age 70, this diversity appears to plummet abruptly. A similar qualitative pattern holds for the CD4 T memory-cell population. The primary question remains whether or not, the loss of diversity is due to a decline in emigration of cells from the thymus or a contraction in total number of cells. [20] In parallel with the parenchymal atrophy, E-rosette-forming cells continuously decrease with age and are progressively replaced by an increasing proportion of 'null' lymphoid cells. These changes appeared to be independent of each other. [21]

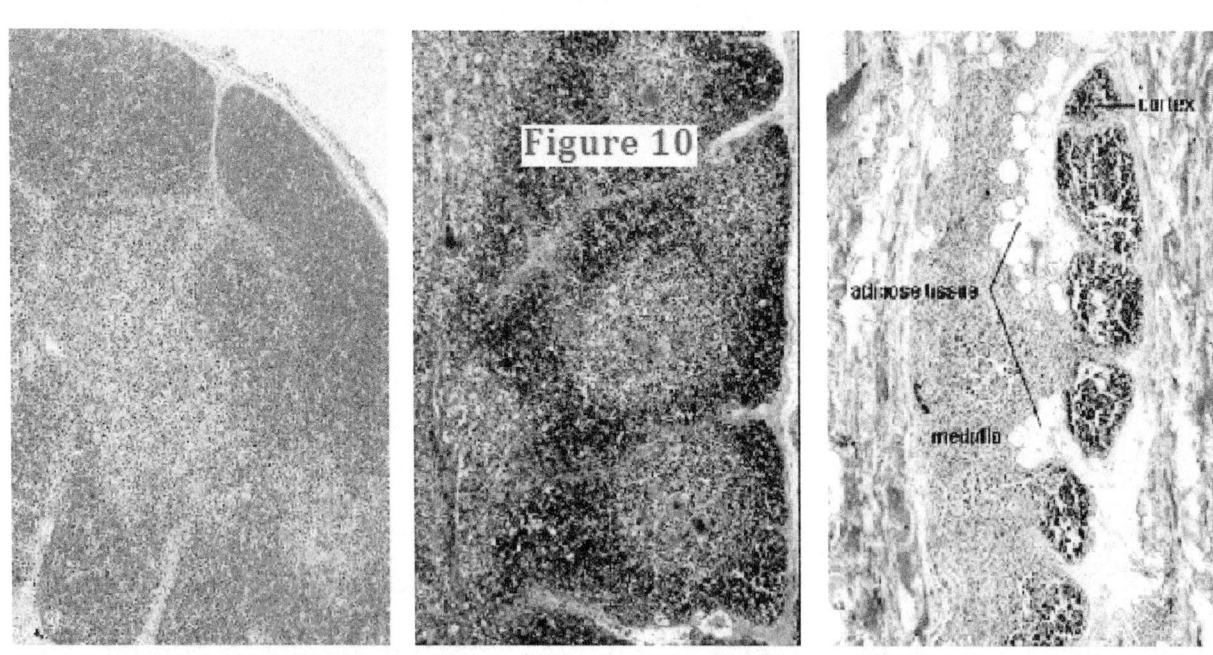

Figure 10

Thymic tissue of human fetus   Thymic tissue of a child   Thymic tissue of adult

Another study suggests that the size of the naive T-cell pool is governed by the output from the thymus and not by replication. This pool contributes cells to the activated/memory T-cell pool whose size can be increased through cell multiplication; both pools together constitute the peripheral T-cell pool. Aging is associated with involution of the thymus leading to a reduction in its contribution to the naive T-cell pool; however, despite this diminished thymic output, there is no significant decline in the total number of T cells in the peripheral T-cell pool. There are, however, considerable shifts in the ratios of both pools of cells, with an increase in the number of activated/memory T-cells and the accumulation in older individuals of cells that fail to respond to stimuli as efficiently as T-cells from younger individuals. [23]

The lymphoid component of the thymus in organotypic culture is primarily presented by low-differentiated CD5(+)-lymphocytes, while mature T and B cells are less abundant. Dipeptide vilon stimulates differentiation of precursors into T-helpers, cytotoxic T lymphocytes, and B cells, while tetrapeptide epithalon stimulates their differentiation towards B cells. Dipeptide vilon acts as an inductor of differentiation of pineal immune cells, which can play an important compensatory role in age-related atrophy of the thymus. Tripeptide vesugen has no effect on differentiation capacity of immune cells of the thymus, but enhances their proliferation potential.[1]

Another interesting study investigated the dynamics and morphology of thymus macrophages in response to thymus involution caused by hyperglycemia.[22] Diabetes' impact on the components of the thymus stroma is largely unknown. The dynamics and morphology of macrophages in the diabetic thymus were investigated by histology, immunohistochemistry, qPCR, electron microscopy and flow cytometry. It was concluded that the thymus involutes rapidly and persistently after the onset of hyperglycemia because of the elevated apoptosis in the thymocytes. These results in an overall increase in macrophage activity in the diabetic thymus in response to the elevated apoptosis of thymocytes produced by hyperglycemia.

Thymic decline in the aged is linked to increased morbidity and mortality in a wide range of clinical settings. Negative consequences of this phenomenon on global health make it of paramount importance to understand the mechanisms driving thymic involution and homeostatic processes across the lifespan. There is growing evidence that thymus tissue is plastic and that the involution process might be therapeutically halted or reversed. [24,25]

Further, in this manual, we discuss current trends in biomedicine in reversing the thymic involution in humans through its regeneration. It updates the progress on the exploitation of thymosuppressive and thymostimulatory pathways using factors such as keratinocyte growth factor, interleukin7 or sex steroid ablation for therapeutic thymus restoration and peripheral immune reconstitution in adults.

Thymic defense of malice and psychic attacks

The terms like "psychic attack" or "venomous harassment" actually cover a broad spectrum of situations in which one individual, the aggressor, deliberately projects a clearly defined malicious intent upon the victim. To differentiate, the intended results of the attack may affect the physical body through disease or death, but the attack itself is aimed at the non-physical planes of the human energy field.

Psychic attacks range in complexity from a very brief, but highly emotionally charged anger or hatred with a "wish" for some clearly defined negative consequence, to the very elaborate, ritualistic practice of malicious sorcery. Although the practice of psychic attack covers such a broad spectrum, the principles of psychic self-defense are much more universal. Once you have "mastered" the techniques of psychic self-defense, and in the absence of some vastly superior power, the application of basic psychic self defense will work.

The psychic attack constitutes of the five elements: desire, intent, alignments, ritual, and expectation:

■ The DESIRE aspect is based not only on the aggressor's malicious impulse, but on the motive for the attack, as well. Since psychic attacks are based solely on the aggressor's perception of a person or situation, the attack and the motive may have no basis in fact. This does not prevent the aggressor from feeling justified, if not benevolent, in initiating the attack. Because of this "perception factor," many victims either never realize that they have been targeted, or fail to accurately grasp the motive or the severity of such an attack. In only the ugliest motives of maliciousness are psychic attacks totally unprovoked.

■ The INTENT aspect is the clearly defined result or outcome of the attack. The more forethought and clearly defined programming the aggressor completes, the more successful the assault will become, lacking any adequate defenses by the intended victim. To be most effective, the attack should include such programming as the time and place of the assault to produce maximum vulnerability, the victim's point of vulnerability, the programmed objective and method of execution, and the post-attack dissipation of the energy or projected thought form.

■ In the ALIGNMENT aspect, the aggressor must eliminate any internal conflict within himself/herself regarding the intended act. Internal conflict or stimuli, as it relates to psychic attack, is normally generated when there is a moral issue associated with the intent. The purest act of magic will manifest with the greatest expectation of success when there is no internal conflict. Any internal conflict will have a proportionately negative effect on the aggressor's chances of success.

■ RITUAL is the aspect that generates and focuses the power necessary to accomplish the attack. Rituals can be as simple or as complex as the practitioner chooses or requires, but the function is always the same. Frequently, in the creation of a psychic attack, the aggressor uses a likeness of the intended victim in the form of a doll called a "poppet".

■ Having now completed all of the steps of the attack, the aggressor has only to watch and wait with EXPECTATION for the psychic assault to take its course. In association with the psychic attack, this is a good time for the aggressor to set up whatever protection is required in the event that the victim successfully repels the attack and the attack is turned back against the aggressor. This is a mistake that many who practice psychic attack make, thinking no one would dare oppose them or even have the power to oppose them. This mistake can be fatal.

What the thymus has to do with all above? Like the assassin plotting the attack on his next physical victim, the psychic attacker plots the attack on his intended victim. In order for the psychic attack to be successful, it must penetrate the victim's consciousness and implant itself deep within the subconscious, where it alters the victim's "illusion of reality." Attached and rooted deep within the subconscious, the psychic attack spins its web around the victim's very thoughts and beliefs and immune system, altering and disrupting normal patterns in such a subversive way that the psychic attacks presence is almost imperceptible. By the time the attacks effects become noticeable, the damage is well established and advanced. The carefully programmed attack is now one with you.

How the attack penetrates the subconscious and establishes itself depends on the victim's vulnerabilities. The entire human system is a complex bio-electro-magnetic field. The psychic attack is a projected thought, an energy form carrying a magnetized imprint of a malignant pattern programmed to disrupt a specific energy pattern within the intended victim's subconscious. It really does not matter how the attack penetrates the subconscious, its presence by whatever means is sufficient. Psychic attacks are always the product of some form of suggestion. Suggestion simply means that a message has bypassed the conscious mind and was planted directly in to the subconscious. This is the entire basis of subliminal programming for weight loss, to quit smoking, become motivated, or overcome a terminal disease.

But suggestion is a two-edged sword. The subconscious mind (the limbic system) does not analyze or judge incoming data. It simply acts on the information that is programmed and imprinted within it.

Getting through it requires a knowledge in a whole discipline, or even more than one discipline. The auric layers are actually egg-shaped, luminous energy fields that completely encapsulate the physical body in ever-expanding layers of higher frequency energy fields. Each layer can be defined by location, color, brightness, form, density, fluidity, and function. The layers are connected to the organs and biological systems of the body through a series of energy vortices called "chakras". The "auric layers" correspond to the chakras. Figure 11 shows the location of each chakra and the associated organ- districts.

Chakra One - the base or the "Root" stands for sexual energy, regeneration and creative drive.

Chakra Two - the "Sacral Endocrine System," stands for the emotional aspects of human consciousness, purification, metabolism, and coping with stress.

Chakra Three - the "Solar Plexus," stands for the sympathetic nervous system and the adrenal glands, body energy, circulation and general mood; also intellectual thought and linear reckoning.

Chakra Four - the 'Heart" stands for the thymus, and is associated with love, both individual as well as humanitarian.

Chakra Five - the "Throat and Thyroid"- stands for the higher will and the power of the spoken word, ability to speak out truth, and take responsibility for actions.

Chakra Six - the "Third Eye" - the pituitary gland - visualization and psychic powers.

Figure 11

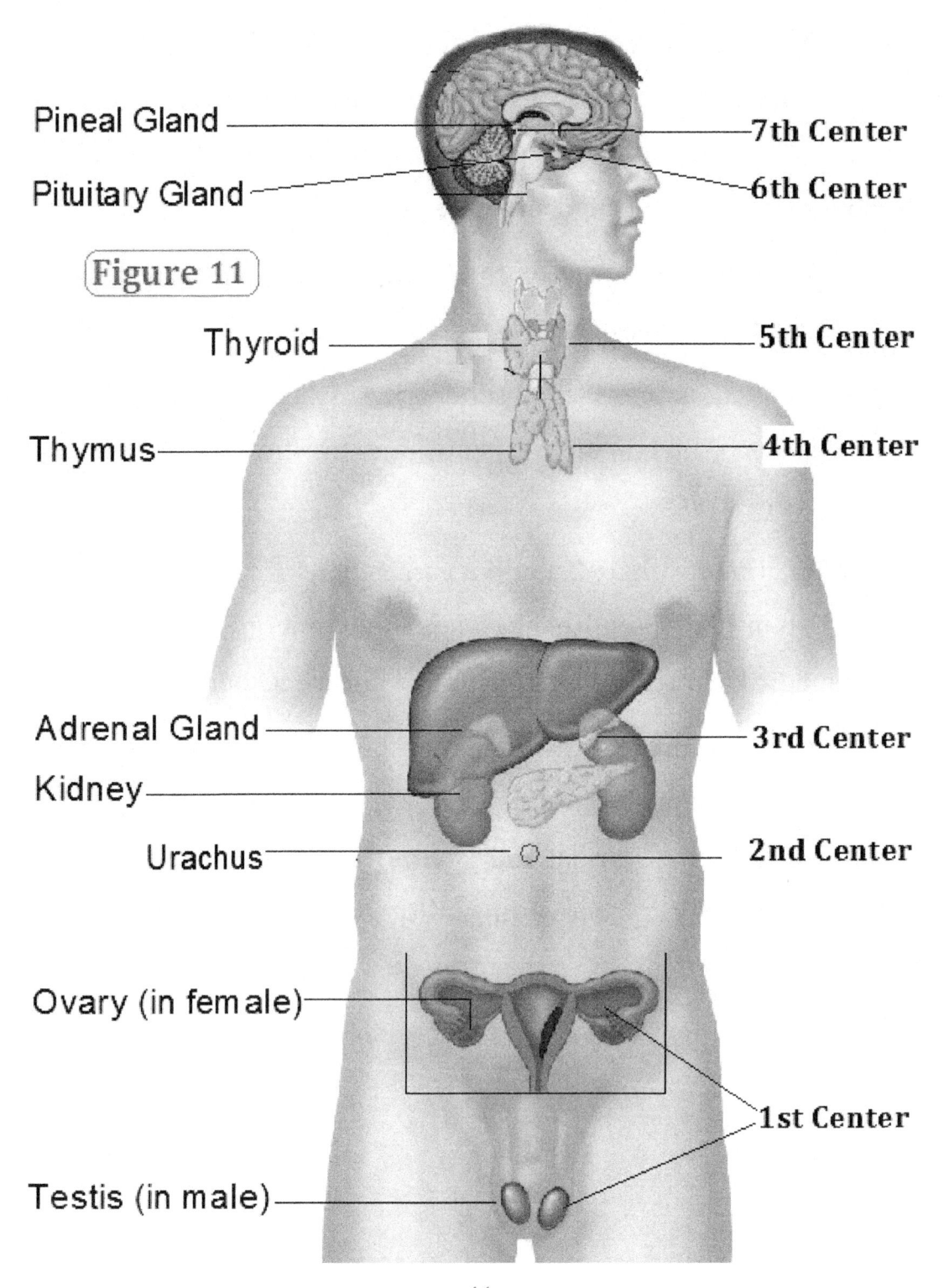

- Pineal Gland — 7th Center
- Pituitary Gland — 6th Center
- Thyroid — 5th Center
- Thymus — 4th Center
- Adrenal Gland — 3rd Center
- Kidney
- Urachus — 2nd Center
- Ovary (in female) — 1st Center
- Testis (in male)

Chakra Seven - the "Crown" - the pineal gland - connects to our higher self as well as the other world and the Divine. It is our connection with the higher universal mind, and the integration of our spiritual and physical makeup.

As seen from the **Figure 10**, the thymus is the central chakra and stands for the balance of the rest. It is the "heart" or "core chakra."

Any incoming psychic attack must attempt to access your subconscious, and thus your conscious reality or your physical body through one or more of these channels. The object of the psychic attack is to disrupt the natural harmony within your body and your illusion of reality. In some cases, by creating a disruption within the body, the aggressor either intends to inflict pain, suffering, or death. In other cases, the aggressor intends to create a disruption in the harmony and continuity of life's natural events. In the most severe cases, the aggressor may actually intend to create such disruption and exert such control over you as to actually "own" you (steal your soul.)

It is important to understand that the creation of these advanced forms of psychic attack are generally well beyond the range of the average person. So, how to protect yourself from "evil"? One of the most common techniques if the "visualized protection" technique. This employs Chakras 7 and 6 and is about comforting yourself with an elevated spirit of goodness, good will, and security that is above the attack. This is very much like affirmations, especially those affirmations used to treat terminal disease. Using the sufficient emotional power you imprint the desired reality on the subconscious live. Any system lacking sufficient power to reach and affect the subconscious mind fails. It's that simple.

The thymus stands for the power of emotions, luck, and immunity. The thymic chakra or connects the emotions of Divine love, compassion, truth and forgiveness. This is the area of the etheric heart. It is sometimes called the *Seat of the Soul.* You must charge and reinforce that armor. Raise your emotional level, directing all the power generated into those shields. Feel the power flowing through you and around you. Feel the shields come up and slam into place. Hear them lock into perfect position. Experience the moment. Feel it, practice it, memorize it, empower it, and reinforce it. The subconscious has the power to do that. But it must be programmed to respond instantly to your thought command. This also involves the Chakra 3.

There is not much to do than to love: love your parents (urachus, standing for the Chakra-2, projects the place of the umbilical connection between you and your mother), and love your family, your job, your enemies. Love is the utmost powerful immunological modulator.

Monitoring thymus

The majority of studies on thymus are through the animal-models. In humans, monitoring thymus function is typically limited to noninvasive technology, including imaging of thymus size with chest-computed tomography or glucose-analog uptake with positron emission tomography.[26, 27]

Peripheral monitoring of thymic output in humans is restricted to surrogate marker analysis of naïve T-cell populations in the blood. Naïve T-cells can be identified by flow cytometry-based immunophenotyping of CD45RA, the high molecular weight isoform of the tyrosine phosphatase CD45, and coexpression of CD62 ligand (CD62L; L-selectin). However, the identification of naïve T-cells with this method can be complicated by memory T-cells (typically CD45RO-positive), which revert to expressing CD45RA, or shedding CD62L by naïve cells after sample cyropreservation.[28, 29]

Given these complications, *Douek et al (2000)* developed a molecular assay that specifically identifies recent thymic emigrants (RTEs) by targeting a DNA byproduct of thymopoiesis.[30] The majority of developing thymocytes rearranges their TCR α genes, which creates an episomal circle of the excised, intervening TCR δ locus. The TCR δ DNA forms what is called a signal joint TCR excision circle (sjTREC). A specialized, real-time PCR reaction was adapted to quantify this nonreplicating circle of DNA in naïve T-cells. Thus, the frequency of molecular sjTREC in a given population of peripheral blood leukocytes is proportional to the degree of thymic output of naïve T- cells.

Another set of arrays monitoring human thymus includes the stimulation of lymphocyte proliferation, Multi-step fractionation by solvent extractions, gel filtrations, ion-exchange chromatography, magnetic resonance imaging (MRI), and of course, the identification of viable CD4+.

CD4+ recent thymic emigrants comprise a clinically and immunologically important T cell population that indicates thymic output and that is essential for maintaining a diverse αβ–T cell receptor (TCR) repertoire of the naive CD4+ T cell compartment. Protein tyrosine kinase 7 (PTK7) is a novel marker for human CD4+ RTEs. Consistent with their recent thymic origin, human PTK7+ RTEs contains higher levels of signal joint TCR gene excision circles and were more responsive to interleukin (IL)-7 compared with PTK7− naive CD4+ T-cells, and rapidly decreased after complete thymectomy. Importantly, CD4+ RTEs proliferates less and produces less IL-2 and interferon-γ than PTK7− naive CD4+ T cells after αβ-TCR/CD3 and CD28 engagement. This immaturity in CD4+ RTE effector function may contribute to the reduced CD4+ T-cell immunity observed in contexts in which CD4+ RTEs predominate, such as in the fetus and neonate or after immune reconstitution. The ability to identify viable CD4+

RTEs by PTK7 staining should be useful for monitoring thymic output in both healthy individuals and in patients with genetic or acquired CD4+ T-cell immunodeficiencies. [31]

The monoclonal antibodies should prove useful for separating and classifying subpopulations of stromal cells and also for monitoring changes in the thymic architecture in different thymic pathologies. Some of the monoclonal antibodies and also OKM1 are identified keratin-negative cells within Hassall's corpuscles, which implies that there are macrophages associated with these structures. [32]

Striking data was presented on the use of human growth hormone (rHGH) and its impact on thymus reconstitution in people with HIV. Marked increases in thymus mass at six months were noted, beyond what have been seen using anti-HIV therapy alone. This increase was sustained over the course of rHGH therapy and correlated with an increase in naive T-cells, most notably naive CD4 cells - suggesting that the thymus is functioning properly and contributing to new T-cells. The development of new, naive T-cells is critical to true immune restoration. [33]

Thymus in stress and distress

Stress disrupts the homeostatic balance of the immune system and causes acute thymic involution through physiologic conditions, such as malnutrition, emotional distress, or pathological conditions, like infection, disease, clinical cancer treatments, preparative regimens for bone marrow transplant. Unfortunately, the thymus is sensitive to acute stress-induced atrophy and is often referred to as a *"barometer of stress"* for the body. Acute thymic atrophy can therefore contribute to the development of a less-diverse, oligoclonal peripheral T-cell repertoire and constricted host immunity. Currently, there are no treatments available to protect against acute thymic atrophy or accelerate recovery.

Acute stress-induced thymic atrophy is a complication from many environmental stressors as well, in which transient reduction in thymus function persists until the physiological stressor is removed. The effects of malnutrition, starvation, and alcoholism have a negative impact on human thymopoiesis. [34, 35]

Many lessons can be learned from the study of thymopoiesis across the lifespan and chronic age-induced thymic involution to facilitate our understanding of cytokine regulation in the setting of acute stress-induced thymic atrophy.

Members of the IL-6 cytokine gene family are increased with age in human thymus tissue.[36] The key IL-6 cytokine gene family members, leukemia inhibitory factor (LIF), IL-6, and Oncostatin M (OSM), are thymosuppressive and play a key role in actively mediating thymus involution. These cytokines are present in the thymic microenvironment and are produced by thymic epithelial cells, which are also capable of producing other immunoregulatory cytokines such as IL-1, IL-3, IL-7, and Tumor growth factor (TGF)-β. [37]

LIF and IL-6 are potent, proinflammatory cytokines that play an integral role in inflammatory responses, such as is observed in LPS-induced acute thymus atrophy. LIF, IL-6, and OSM signal through the common gp130 subunit to the IL-6R family, which is expressed ubiquitously on thymocytes and on thymic epithelium. The IL-6 cytokine family members are acutely thymosuppressive and play a negative role in thymus atrophy induced by lipopolysaccharide (LPS). LIF, IL-6, and OSM are mediators of both LPS-induced and stress-induced thymic atrophy. [38]

LIF is a known activator of the hypothalamic-pituitary-adrenal (HPA) axis. LIF is unable to induce thymic atrophy when corticosterone production is blocked by the synthesis inhibitor metyrapone or by adrenalectomy, indicating that the mechanism of action of LIF is corticosteroid-dependent.[39, 40] Thymic epithelial cells possess all of the enzymes necessary for steroidogenesis and produce small amounts of corticosterone, which at normal physiological levels modulate thymocyte activation thresholds for proper positive and negative selection. LIF acts as a thymosuppressive cytokine via intrathymic and systemic mechanisms and may be an effector pathway of chronic and acute thymic involution.[41]

In summary, IL-6 cytokine family members mediate their both normal and thymosuppressive effects via the thymic stroma. The intrathymic production of corticosteroids induced by LIF is a specific example of a stromal-mediated response.[42] Ablation of STAT3, an intracellular signaling molecule involved in the activation of many IL-6 family cytokine receptors, specifically from thymic epithelial cells, results in severe thymic atrophy caused by loss of thymic epithelial cells as well as thymocytes.[43] More research is needed to identify the relative contribution of cytokine signaling through thymocytes or thymic epithelial cells in the role of stress-induced thymic atrophy. Regardless, these data and other observations support a new paradigm, in which cytokines act as thymosuppressors in settings of stress-induced acute thymic atrophy.

The thymus monitors and regulates energy flow throughout the body. Whenever an imbalance occurs, it rebalances the energy. The thymus is the first organ to be affected by stress, whether it is physical stress - infection, disease - or mental stress. It is the link between mind and body.

The thymus is influenced by an individual's physical environment, social environment, food, posture, and emotional attitudes. Thinking about something unpleasant will weaken the thymus, while thinking about someone you love will strengthen it. The negative emotional - weakening - states are hate, envy, suspicion, and fear. The positive emotional states are love, faith, trust, courage and gratitude. We call these latter states thymus qualities.

Chronic physical or emotional stress activates the HPA axis to induce production of the stress hormones, glucocorticoids (GCs). Glucocorticoids cause abrupt thymus involution and result in a failure or breakdown in immunological tolerance. As a result autoreactive T-cells are escaped from thymus microenvironment which ensures self/non-self education and selection of mature T-cells before being exported to the periphery. Though regulatory T-cells are present in the circulation, they are unable to suppress the autoreactive T-cells from initiating the destruction of β-cells and the subsequent development of autoimmune diseases, like lupus, or type 1 diabetes. The destruction of β-cells can be mediated by various mechanisms including Fas-FasL, perforin/granzymes, reactive oxygen species, and cytokines (e.g., IL- 1β, IFN-γ).[44]

Leptin

Leptin is one of the most important adipose-derived 16-kDa protein hormones (Figure 12). It plays a key role in regulating energy intake and energy expenditure, including appetite, hunger and metabolism.

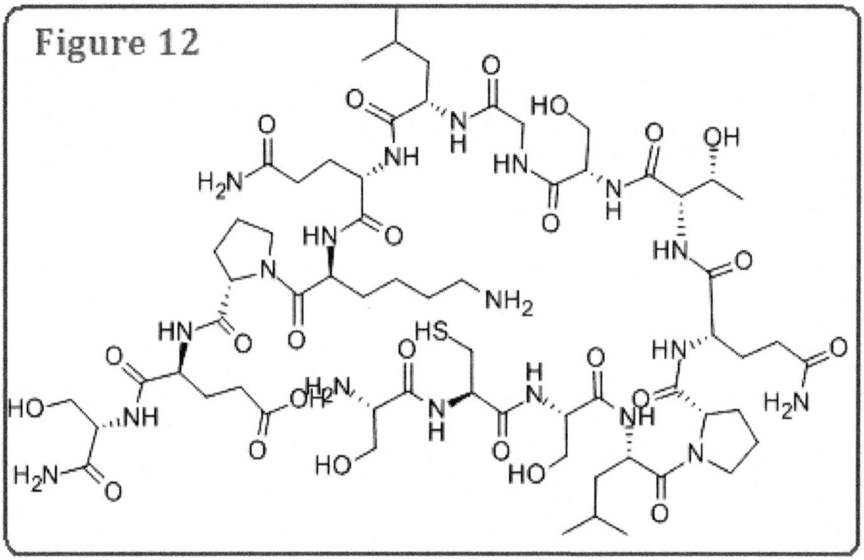

Figure 12

Leptin is primarily produced by adipocytes and has many roles in the neuroendocrine and reproductive systems. It is known for its role in satiety and feeding behavior. But leptin is more than a satiety hormone. It has structural similarities to class I cytokines (IL-6 gene family), and its receptor has structural similarities to the class I cytokine receptor gp130 subunit. For this reason, leptin is cross-classified as a cytokine.[45]

A role for leptin in modulating immunity was first speculated by the observance of suppressed cell-mediated immunity, chronic thymic atrophy, and decreased numbers of lymphocytes in ob/ob and db/db mice. The impact of leptin on cells of the immune system continues to be an emerging area of investigation, with several functions of leptin in innate and adaptive immunity already identified. [46, 47]

Leptin influences many cells important to innate immunity, such as dendritic cells, macrophages, neutrophils, and NK cells. Leptin also modulates CD4 Th cell cytokine production, favoring a Th1 response versus Th2 response, and preferentially promotes naïve T-cell proliferation and inhibits memory T cell proliferation.[48] Leptin also plays a role in autoimmune disorders. [49]

Leptin has been found to constrain the proliferation of T regulatory cells, thymic-derived cells charged with maintaining peripheral tolerance. It acts as a pleiotropic mediator in a wide-range of biological systems (neuroendocrine, immune). [50]

Thymus atrophy associated with leptin deficiency or leptin receptor deficiency has long been an indicator that leptin may play a role in normal thymopoiesis. It has been discussed whether thymic atrophy from leptin deficiency is a result of the stress seen from metabolic and hormonal dysregulation, as opposed to direct effects in the thymus. *Palmer et al (2006)* shed light on this issue by addressing the following questions: does leptin receptor deficiency result in a cellular defect of lymphocytes or thymic stromal cells, and is thymic atrophy simply mediated by the metabolic defects of leptin receptor-deficient mice, such as elevated corticosterone levels? [51]

Through a series of experiments using bone marrow chimeras (BMC) in between db/db mice and their lean heterozygous littermates (db/+) the authors revealed that a cellular defect of the thymus stroma or an environmental effect mediated by corticosterone and/or other metabolic factors was the cause of the observed thymus atrophy. Thus, environmental factors play a large role in the chronic thymic atrophy, in which corticosterone is a likely mediator. In agreement with these observations, other studies have found that exogenous leptin treatment is unable to boost thymus cellularity of healthy, wild-type mice. [52, 53]

How leptin protects against stress-induced thymic atrophy? Leptin has been reported to be thymostimulatory in settings of thymus stress. It has therapeutic potential in the lipopolysaccharide (LPS) stress model of acute thymic atrophy. Leptin is able to significantly blunt the LPS-induced thymus weight loss with a trend toward increased cellularity. [52] It also completely protects against the LPS-induced loss of mTREC/mg thymus.[54]

Here we conclude that leptin as a novel, thymostimulatory agent that can protect against endotoxin-induced acute thymic atrophy.

Relaxin

Relaxin is a peptide of the insulin step-family and consists of seven peptides of high structural but low sequence similarity; relaxin-1 (RLN1), 2 (RLN2) and 3 (RLN3), and the insulin-like (INSL) peptides, INSL3, INSL4, INSL5 and INSL6 (Figure 13). In the female, it is produced by the corpus luteum of the ovary, the breast and during pregnancy, through the placenta, chorion, and decidua. In the male, it is produced in the prostate and is present in human semen.

Figure 13

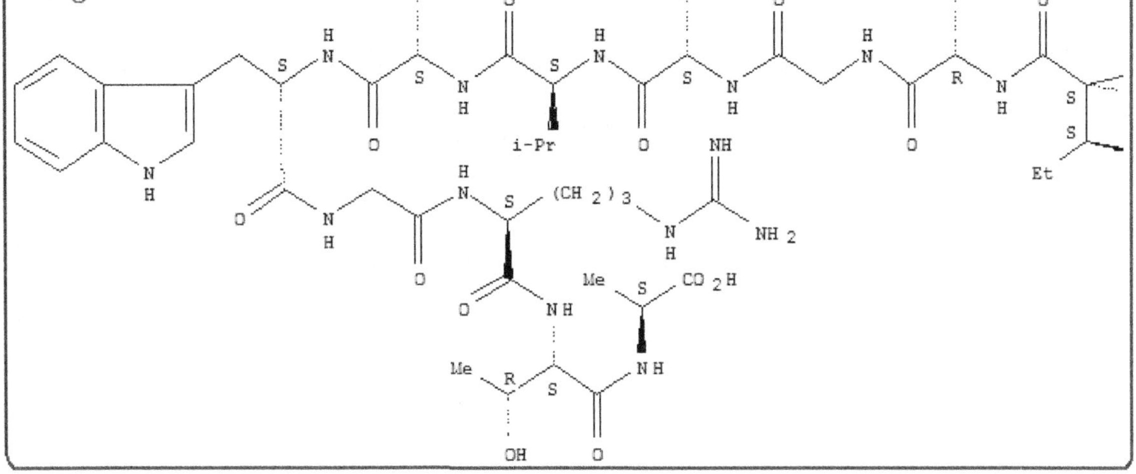

Relaxin was discovered more than 75 years prior to the identification of the receptors that mediate its actions. There has been a slow emergence in understanding its role, with it being denoted initially as a hormone of pregnancy. The effects of relaxin are most well-described during the female reproductive cycle and pregnancy. However, many other physiological roles have been identified for relaxin, including cardiovascular and neuropeptide functions and an ability to induce the matrix metalloproteinases, so it is clear that relaxin is not exclusively a hormone of pregnancy but has a much wider role in vivo.

The recent de-orphanisation of four receptors LGR7, LGR8, GPCR135 (SALPR) and GPCR142 (GPR100) that respond to and bind at least one of the three forms of relaxin identified to date, allows dissection of this system to determine the precise role of each receptor and enable the identification of new targets for treatment of numerous disease states.

Relaxin-3, the most recently identified member of the relaxin peptide family, is produced by GABAergic projection neurons in the nucleus incertus (NI), in the pontine periventricular gray. Relaxin-3 is a modulator of stress responses, metabolism, arousal and behavioral activation. Yet, a definitive role remains elusive due to discrepancies between models and a propensity to investigate pharmacological effects over endogenous function.

Relaxin has the potential to be useful for the treatment of scleroderma, fibrosis, in orthodontics and to facilitate embryo implantation in humans. One of the riddles of fibromyalgia and myofascial pain is relaxin, that make the muscles and collagen relax. The antiarthritic effect of the relaxin is also well established. [55] Relaxin antagonists may act as contraceptives or prevent the development of breast cancer metastases. Recent research has added considerable knowledge to the signaling pathways activated by relaxin, which will aid our understanding of how relaxin produces its effects.

Both during phylogeny and ontogeny the thymus appears as a nodal point between the two major systems of cell-to-cell signaling, the neuroendocrine and immune systems. The neuroendocrine polypeptide precursors play a dual role in T-cell selection played by the thymic repertoire. Thymic neuroendocrine-related polypeptides are a source of self-antigens which are presented by the major histocompatibility system of the thymic epithelium. The intrathymic T-cell education to neuroendocrine self-antigens is not strictly superimposible to the antigen presentation by dedicated presenting cells.[56]

Yet, little is known about the role of relaxin in modulating cell-mediated immunity, and acute or chronic thymic atrophy. The only existing putative relations are speculated through the passage illustrated in **Figure 14**:

Figure 14: Projective Thymic-Relaxin Pathway

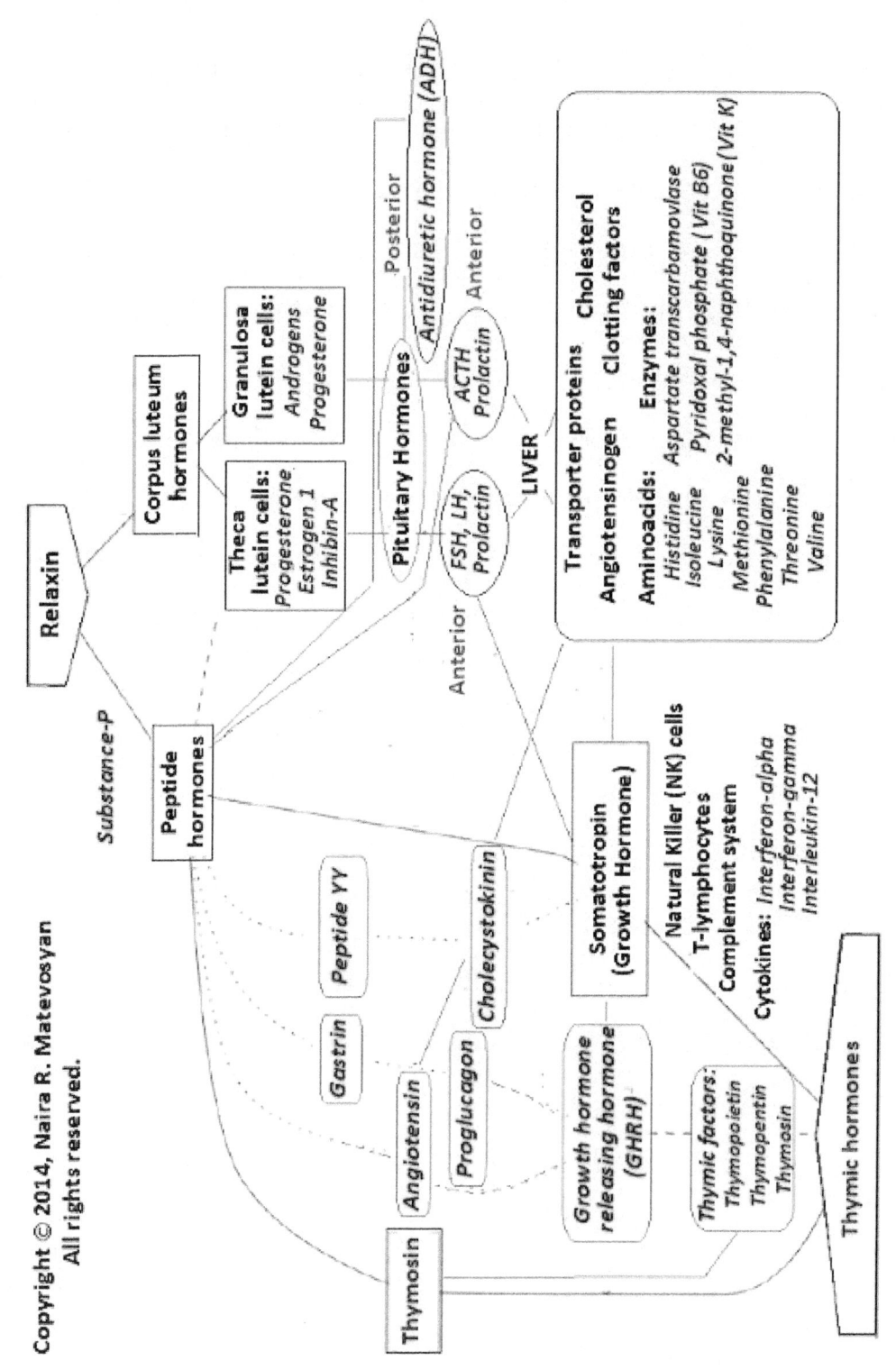

Thymus and sex hormones

The thymus is a temporary organ, but it plays vital roles when it's active - helping the body protect itself against autoimmunity. It plays a central role in the lymphatic and endocrine systems. It is in charge of the development and maintenance of immunological competence.

In fetus and throughout childhood, the thymus is instrumental in the production and maturation of T-lymphocytes or T cells, produces and secretes thymosin, a hormone necessary for T-cell development and production. Unlike most organs, the thymus is at its largest in children. It shrinks after puberty, fortunately, having produced all of the T- cells by puberty.

T-cell progenitor cells (stem cells) originating in bone marrow migrate to the thymus where they undergo a remarkable maturation process. Here, the immature T-cells (thymocytes) differentiate into different classes, including T-helper cells and cytotoxic T-cells. Afterwards, the cells undergo a critical selection process in which only T-cells capable of recognizing non-self antigens displayed on the surface of "professional" antigen-presenting cells (e.g. macrophages, dendritic cells) are allowed to survive. As much as 98% of the T-cells fail this selection process and are degraded. The rest migrate to peripheral sites throughout the body to perform their specific immunological roles.

Thymic involution is a process directed by the increased circulation of sex hormones, gonadal steroids. Proportional to thymic size, thymic activity (T cell output) is most active before puberty. Upon atrophy, the size and activity are dramatically reduced, and the organ is primarily replaced with fat. Chemical or physical castration of an adult results in the thymus increasing in size and activity.

Below is the growth dynamics of the thymus:

Newborn ~ 15 grams;

Puberty ~ 35 grams

25 years ~ 25 grams

60 years less than 15 grams

70 years ~ 0 grams

In this chapter, we present the mechanism of sex hormone actions on the thymus, presenting mainly data obtained at the cellular and molecular levels. First, data supporting the "genomic" action via the nuclear sex hormone receptor complexes are as follows:

1) sex hormone receptors and the thymic factor (thymulin) are co-localized in thymic epithelial cells, but not in T-cells;

2) production/expression of thymic factors (thymulin, thymosin alpha-1) are remarkably inhibited by sex hormone treatment; and

3) sex hormones cause changes in T-cell subpopulations in the thymus.

Secondly, data indicating the "non-genomic" action of sex hormones via a membrane signal-generating mechanism are as follows:

1) the proliferation/maturation of thymic epithelial cells is mediated through protein kinase C activity introduced by sex hormones;

2) sex hormones directly influence DNA synthesis and cdc2 kinase (cell cycle-promoting factor) activity.[57]

As an ob-gyn doctor, I am more interested in clinical manifestations of residual thymic pathology in reproductive health of women. It is known that secretion of thymulin follows a circadian rhythm, peaking during the night, just opposite to circadian rhythm of the glucocorticoids (GCs). GCs exert the profound anti-inflammatory and immunosuppressive activity. They may be associated with a topical and systemic adverse effects caused by prolonged or chronic activation of the HPA axis or by continuous high-dose treatment.

Metabolic correlations of GCs and gonadal steroids with thymic function are poorly understood. GCs participate in ovarian and testicular functions. GCs suppress both gonadotropin-releasing hormone (GnRH) and gonadotropins secretion inhibiting testosterone and estradiol production by testis and ovary, respectively. Psychological stress can lead to reproductive suppression. In males, decreased serum testosterone (T) is one of the first signs of stress. During the excessive exposure to GCs apoptosis is initiated in Leydig cells, the preeminent source of testosterone. Humans exposed to prolonged stress respond with the inhibition of luteinising hormone (LH) release and blocked ovulation.

Several studies suggest that thymus is the primary sex hormone-responsive organ. The thymus is the major target of estrogens in the immune system. Ovariectomy reduces serum estrogen levels and results in enlargement of the female thymus.[58] Other studies demonstrate that the thymus undergoes involution after testosterone and estrogen treatment, but not progesterone, following gonadectomy.[59]

Interestingly, in thymomas, once thymomagenesis is set up, tumor cells lose their sensitivity to sexual hormones, resulting in automatic differentiation and/ or proliferation according to the process programmed by the dominant gene *Tsr-1*.

Thymus weight and cellular composition are very sensitive to changes in androgen status. The thymus gland of male animals is enlarged under conditions of androgen deficiency.[60]

Thymus and maternal-fetal immunology

During the pregnancy the thymus shrinks dramatically. A specific study suggests that whilst the thymic cortex involutes, the medulla enlarges and rearranges to create a microenvironment containing increased numbers of mature thymocytes (Figure 15). It is suggested that these recently derived T-cells may contribute to the unique populations of cells with suppressive function that appear during pregnancy, and thereby contribute to the immune suppression of the mother to paternal and fetal antigens. In addition, the pregnancy-associated cortical involution of the thymus may reflect the deletion of clones with potential reactivity to paternal and/or fetal antigens.[61]

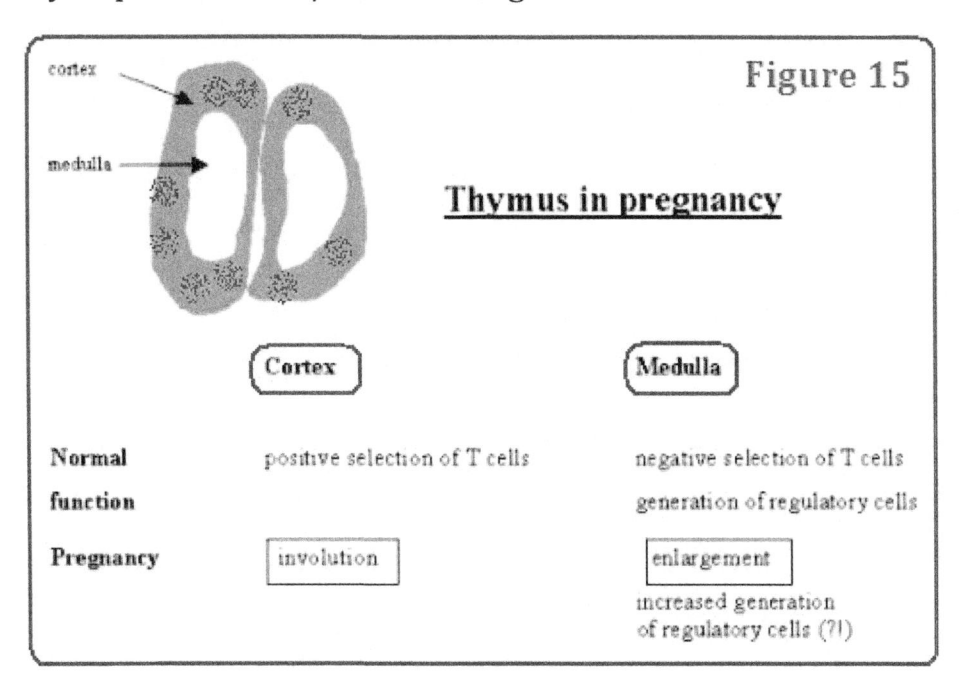

Figure 15

Thymus in pregnancy

	Cortex	Medulla
Normal function	positive selection of T cells	negative selection of T cells; generation of regulatory cells
Pregnancy	involution	enlargement; increased generation of regulatory cells (?!)

One of the long-standing enigmas of reproductive biology is why the fetus is not rejected by the mother's immune system. Many explanations for this phenomenon have been proposed and tested, including the idea of paternal antigen sequestration and reduced MHC expression, the possibility of local immune changes in the uterus, and a potential maternal shift from Th1 to Th2 immune responses. [62]

Although each of these mechanisms appears to play some role in protection of the fetus from the maternal immune system, none has been directly shown to be required. It now appears that pregnancy may in fact have many redundant mechanisms acting both systemically and at the maternal–fetal interface to protect the fetus from the mother's immune system.

One particularly interesting effect of pregnancy on maternal immune system is a general blockade of lymphocyte development. This blockade manifests itself grossly in the form of thymic involution and bone marrow involution. Involution of the thymus has long been recognized to occur during pregnancy in a number of species and human and may be mimicked by the administration of the female sex hormones estrogen (E) and progesterone (P), although the relative contributions of the two hormones are controversial. Although the functional importance of pregnancy-induced thymic involution remains unknown, the fact that it has been observed in all mammals has led to the speculation that reduced or altered output of mature T-cells by the thymus could be an important component of maternal immune regulation. It also has been reported that bone marrow, the site of B lymphocyte development, undergoes an involution process similar to that occurring in the thymus during pregnancy. The result is a specific block to B-cell development that can be replicated by E + P treatment.

As the major hormone of pregnancy, progesterone is an obvious candidate mediator for pregnancy-associated phenomena. Progesterone receptor (PR) regulates virtually all aspects of female reproduction, including ovulation, uterine decidualization, sexual lordosis behavior, and mammary gland development.

Thymic involution in pregnancy occurs in later pregnancy and reaches a maximum at parturition. After childbirth the involuted thymus regenerates. Lactation has an inhibitory influence on the regeneration. The possible significance of the thymic changes relate to the adrenocortical activity. Histologically the cortex exhibits prominent alterations during the involution and regeneration. The pattern of depletion and repopulation of lymphocytes in the cortex is similar to that in other types of acute involution. [63]

Thymus, prolactin, and the growth hormone

Intrathymic T-cell differentiation is under the control of thymic microenvironment, which acts on maturing thymocytes via membrane as well as soluble products. Increasing data show that this process can be modulated by prolactin (PRL) and growth hormone (GH), largely secreted by the pituitary gland.

Both PRL and GH stimulate the secretion of thymulin, a thymic hormone produced by thymic epithelial cells. Conversely, low levels of circulating thymulin parallel hypopituitary states. Interestingly, the enhancing effects of GH on thymulin seem to be mediated by insulinlike growth factor (IGF-1) since they can be abrogated with anti-IGF-1 or anti-IGF-l-receptor antibodies. The influence of PRL and GH on the thymic epithelium is pleiotropic: PRL enhances in vivo the expression of high-molecular-weight cytokeratins and stimulates in vitro TEC proliferation, an effect that is shared by GH and IGF-1.

Differentiating T-cells are also targets for the intrathymic action of PRL and GH. PRL may regulate the maintenance of thymocyte viability during the double-positive stage of thymocyte differentiation.

Injections of GH into aging mice increase total thymocyte numbers and the percentage of CD3-bearing cells, as well as the Concanavalin-A mitogenic response and IL-6 production by thymocytes. Interestingly, similar findings are observed in animals treated with IGF-1. Lastly, the thymic hypoplasia observed in dwarf mice can be reversed with GH treatment. Another randomized trial confirms that GH is an under-appreciated but important regulator of T-cell development that can reverse age-related declines in thymopoiesis in rodents.[64]

In keeping with the data summarized earlier is the detection of receptors for PRL and GH on both thymocytes and thymic epithelial cells. Importantly, recent studies indicate that both cell types can produce PRL and GH intrathymically. Similarly, production of IGF-1 and expression of a corresponding receptor has also been demonstrated.

PRL may participate in two interrelated mechanisms: the regulation of peripheral single-positive cells and the maintenance of thymocyte viability during the double-positive stage of intrathymic differentiation.[65]

These data strongly indicate that the thymus is physiologically under control of pituitary hormones PRL and GH. In addition to the classical endocrine pathway, paracrine and autocrine circuits are probably implicated in such control.[66]

Breastfeeding

Breastfeeding provides unsurpassed natural nutrition and immunological protection to the newborn and infant. Human breast-milk influences on the infant response to vaccination and thymic gland development. The early positive influences of human breast milk may be a bulwark against chronic disease in later life.

For the fetus and newborn, immunologic defenses are present, but immature. To compensate, the mother's immunoglobulin (Ig) G antibody moves across the placental barrier to provide some protection. After birth, these maternal antibodies wane in the first 6 to 12 months of human life. The neonate and infant can receive additional maternal protection from breast milk, however.

Human breast-milk, and especially the early colostrum, contains measurable levels of leukocytes. Colostrum contains approximately 5×10^6 cells per mL, an amount that decreases tenfold in mature milk. Most of these leukocytes are macrophages and neutrophils, which phagocytose microbial pathogens. Lymphocytes, including T-cells, natural killer cells, and antibody-producing B-cells, make up 10% of the leukocytes in human breast milk. These cells survive passage through the infant's gastrointestinal system where they are absorbed and influence the infant's immune response.

Immature T-cells, known as thymocytes, undergo a selection process in the thymus to remove potentially self-reactive cells. Less than 5% of thymocytes survive this "education" to be released as functionally mature, circulating T-cells. While the clinical significance of thymic size is not known, the central role of the thymus gland in the development of the T-cell repertoire suggests a potential for direct effects of breastfeeding on a crucial organ of the maturing immune system.

Using an ultrasound technique to measure thymic index size, *Hasselbalch et al (1996)* have found that, at the fourth months of age, infants who were breastfed exclusively had significantly larger thymus glands than those who were partially breastfed or formula fed only. [67] A correlation was found between breastfeeding and CD8+ T cells. There was no significant difference in thymic size among the three study groups at birth. A later study by *Thompson et al (2000)* was unable to confirm the findings of *Hasselbalch* by measuring thymic weights at autopsy in infants who died of sudden infant death syndrome. [68]

Later, *Hasselbalch et al (1999)* had ran another study, the in continuum to the previous one, showing that the breast-fed infants have a considerably larger thymus at 4 months than formula-fed infants. In a cohort of 50 infants, all being partially breast-fed when recruited at 8 months, ultrasound assessment of the thymic index (a volume estimate) was performed at both 8 and 10 months of age. At 10 months the thymic index was significantly higher in those still being breast-fed compared to infants who had stopped breast-feeding between 8 and 10 months of age (P=0.05). This difference became more significant when controlled for the influence of infectious diseases (P=0.03). In infants still breast-fed at 10 months there was a significant correlation between the number of breast-feeds per day and their thymic index (P=0.01). The authors concluded that the effect of breast-feeding on thymus size was likely to be caused by immune modulating factors in breast-milk. [69]

Could early consumption of human breast-milk also provide long-term benefits by protecting individuals from chronic diseases later in life? There is enough evidence to suggest that breastfeeding may significantly alter the immune system of the suckling infant. Clues to this early influence are seen in the effects of breastfeeding on thymic size, the antibody response to vaccination, and increased tolerance to breast milk leukocyte antigens. Fundamental changes in the infant's immune system as a result of premature cessation of breastfeeding could lay the groundwork for later dysfunction in the immunologic controls necessary to prevent autoimmune disease or hypersensitivity reactions. [70]

Thymus, fecundity, and fertility

Fecundity is the ability to reproduce. It is the potential reproductive capacity of an individual or population. Whereas, fertility is the natural capability of producing offsprings. Fertility is confounded by various factors, such as nutrition, sexual behavior, culture, instinct, endocrinology, timing, economics, way of life, and emotions.

Lack or absence of fecundity is called sterility; lack or absence of fertility is called infertility. Infertility is a condition that affects a couple and is defined as the lack of conception after an arbitrary period of 12 months, without using any contraception. Infertility (for 12 month or more) after one or more pregnancy episodes (miscarriage, preterm or term birth, or stillbirth) is called secondary infertility. Thus, infecundity can be seen as a primary infertility. The World Health Organization (WHO) defines sterility as an illness, but a vast number of countries do not accept this definition.

An interrelationship between immune and reproductive systems has been postulated, and involves, among others, bidirectional effects between gonads and thymus. However, the scarcity (nearing absence) of the thymus information in human reproductive health scholarship, books and textbooks in obstetrics and gynecology, links to the following reasons: (1) being a temporary organ, the thymus shrinks with puberty and therefore looses (mistakenly though) its importance to be seen in any relations with the HPA axis; and (2) ethical constraints and practical difficulties in conducting studies (other than observational) on the thymus in reproductive aged men and women.

Female fertility can be affected by diseases or dysfunctions of reproductive tract, neuroendocrine system, and immune system. Reproductive autoimmune failure can be associated with overall activation of immune system or with immune system reactions specifically directed against ovarian antigens. Majority of the antiovarian autoantibodies are directed against β-subunit of follicle stimulating hormone (anti-FSH). In female infertility the expansion of cells responding to low-affinity ligands (self-antigen) or anomalies in the deletion of high-affinity autoreactive T-cells leading to autoimmune reactions is a possibility.

Infertility and recurrent spontaneous abortion (RSA) are heterogeneous conditions that have been frequently explained with an immunological pathomechanism. A deeper insight into apparently unexplained infertility and RSA shows increasing evidences supporting both alloimmune and autoimmune mechanisms, in which natural killer (NK) cells and autoantibodies seem to play a relevant role. Successful pregnancy is considered as Th1–Th2 cooperation phenomenon, with a predominantly Th2-type lymphocytes response, together with the emerging role of interleukin (IL)-12, IL-15, and IL-18 and of other unidentified soluble factors dependent on NK cells. Uterine NK cells comprise the largest population at implantation site, and their activity, characteristics, and abundance suggest that they participate at the "decidualization" process that, vice versa, induces NK activation and recruitment in each menstrual cycle. However, NK cell alteration may be associated with impaired pregnancy, and the modulation in the number of circulating NK cells is most likely to be a primary event rather than an active inflammation/drug administration consequence during an inflammatory/autoimmune process, thus playing an important role in the pathogenesis of immunological infertility. [71]

Studies on animal models suggest on the reduced fecundity of parasites due to the thymus-dependent immunological responses in mice.[72] Removal of the thymus retards the growth of the testes in young guinea pigs.[72] Another study defines the thymus factor (TF) to inhibit the binding activity of 125I-hCG to its testicular receptor. The inhibitory effect of TF on hCG binding is dose related, suggesting a modulation function of TF at the testis receptor level.[74]

The reproductive autoimmune failure syndrome was originally described by *Gleicher et al.* in 1987, in women with endometriosis, infertility and increased autoantibodies. [75] Autoimmune mechanisms as well as an increased production of multiple autoantibodies are involved in such infertility disorders as premature ovarian failure (POF), endometriosis, polycystic ovary syndrome (PCOS), unexplained infertility, and repeatedly unsuccessful in vitro fertilization (IVF) attempts and may be responsible for the pathophysiology of preeclampsia or spontaneous abortions. Although not many studies have been performed on humans, the role of cellular immunity in ovarian autoimmunity, in addition to humoral immunity, has been detected both locally in the ovary,[76] as well as in periphery. [77]

The autoimmune-associated infertility might be a polyclonal event characterized by immunological defects at the T-cell level which, similarly to classical autoimmune diseases, may manifest itself in abnormal antibody production. [78, 79] However, due to the technical difficulties in everyday laboratory work, most clinical studies are restricted to detecting serum antibodies in order to define autoimmune activation in a patient.

The thymus performs many roles in immune-related fertility issues. Evidence suggests that the autoimmune regulator gene influences thymic production of ovarian antigens and prevents autoimmune-mediated premature reproductive senescence. Immune-mediated ovarian follicular depletion is a mechanism of infertility in mice. The results have important implications in the pathogenesis of ovarian autoimmune disease in women. Thymic expression of ovarian genes under the autoimmune regulator's (AIRE) control may be critical for preventing ovarian autoimmune disease.[80]

It is also established that treatment of patients with chronic prostatitis is complicated by infertility by microwave (460 MHz) action on the area of the thyroid and thymus glands.[81] T-lymphocyte inhibition by human seminal plasma is due to multiple factors, and reduced amounts of these factors may contribute to the development and/or persistence of sperm autoimmunity in infertile men.[82]

Human thymus has been viewed as the main site of tolerance induction to self-antigens that are specifically expressed by thymic cells and abundant blood-borne self-antigens, whereas tolerance to tissue-restricted self-antigens has been ascribed to extrathymic (peripheral) tolerance mechanisms. However, the phenomenon of promiscuous expression of tissue-restricted self-antigens by medullary thymic epithelial cells has led to a reassessment of the role of central T-cell tolerance in preventing organ-specific autoimmunity. Both genetic and epigenetic mechanisms account for this unorthodox mode of gene expression. This manual informs the alarming need to explore further.

Zinc

Zinc is one of the essential elements required by our body in trace amounts. Zinc was initially found to be an essential element for the growth more than 100 years ago. A central figure in these studies was Dr. Ananda Prasad, a hematologist, who found that low zinc levels in blood were casually related to a rare condition of dwarfism, testicular retardation, and susceptibility to infections in a group of patients who, although not genetically related, were alike in having a diet that produced zinc deficiency.

Moderate deficiency of zinc has been associated with numbers of disorders, such as sickle cell anemia, kidney problems, gastral-intestinal diseases, menstrual dysfunction, and many others. Zinc deficiency is one of the causes of altered responses of the immune system. Zinc is considered essential for generating cell-mediated responses. In addition to combining with thymic hormone to form the biologically active thymic hormone molecule, even a mild reduction of circulating zinc levels is associated with reduced T-cell production of cytokines. Animal studies have reported a 30-80% reduction in the function of the immune system when exposed to moderate zinc deficiencies.

Zinc nourishes the thymus, and rejuvenates it. Zinc deficiency results in decline of the thymic function and even in thymic atrophy. This effect is more common in older adults who suffer from nutrient deficiency. Zinc supplementation in older adults has been noted to improve the immune response thereby substantiating the role of zinc in the immune function. [83]

Causes of Zinc Deficiency:

- Vegetarian diets (phytates in plant foods inhibits zinc)
- Low red meat consumption
- Little or no seafood consumption
- Dieting, especially high carbohydrate diets
- Copper toxicity
- Low stomach acid
- Digestive disorders
- Aging, especially if you are over 45

Signs of Zinc Deficiency:

- White spots on your fingernails
- Menstrual irregularities
- Lack of appetite
- Alteration in taste perceptions
- Hair loss

- Poor wounds healing
- Skin breakouts.

Zinc-deficient children also have thymic atrophy and an increased susceptibility to infections. Children with protein-energy malnutrition similarly have thymic atrophy, zinc deficiency, and increased susceptibility to infections. [84]

Meat-based foods high in zinc:	Plant-based foods high in zinc:
- Oyster	- Wheat germ
- Shellfish	- Wheat bran
- Crab-meat	- Pumpkin seeds
- Lobster	- Brown rice
- Turkey	- Beans
- Beef	- Peanuts
- Pork	- Potato

Supplementation to correct zinc deficiencies and boost immunity need not be higher than 15- 30 mg per day. Doses up to 50 mg/ day are considered safe when taken for no more than six months. High doses of zinc however, can displace iron and copper, which can result in elevated cholesterol, anemia and mood alterations. Too much zinc can suppress the immune system. Daily zinc supplement should not exceed 300 mg.

A multiparametric study of the thymus was performed in normal aging mice (12-15 months old) submitted to a mild oral zinc supplementation during 3-6 months. Findings suggested that oral zinc administration stimulates thymus growth and partially restores the micro-environmental as well as lymphoid compartments of the organ. Regarding thymic endocrine function, a significant increase in thymulin levels and a concomitant decrease in plasma thymulin inhibitors were observed, suggesting that the age-related decline of thymic function might at least partially be due to extrinsic factors, such as zinc deficiency. The total number of thymic lymphocytes was consistently increased, without significant changes in CD4/CD8 defined thymocyte subsets. Structural changes of the thymus epithelium were also detected, including the disappearance of epithelial cysts frequently observed in old animals, reappearance of a normal pattern of the thymic epithelial cell network, and a decrease in the extracellular matrix network. [85]

Taken together, these data suggest that aging-related mild zinc deficiency induces some changes in thymus structure and function which can be partially corrected by an oral zinc supplementation.

Thymic rejuvenation and regeneration

A number of organs have the intrinsic ability to regenerate, among them the thymus. Organ regeneration is a promising therapy that can alleviate humans from diseases that have not been yet cured. It is also superior to already existing treatments that utilize exogenous sources to substitute for the organ's lost structure or function(s).

A number of theories have been forwarded to explain the 'thymic menopause' including the possible loss of thymic progenitors or epithelial cells, a diminished capacity to rearrange T-cell receptor genes and alterations in the production of growth factors and hormones. Strategies to improve the consequences of the aging thymus are currently under investigation. Although to date no interventions fully restore thymic function in the aging host, systemic administration of various cytokines and hormones or bone marrow transplantation have resulted in increased thymic activity and T-cell output with age.[23]

Endogenous thymic regeneration is a crucial function that allows for renewal of immune competence after stress, infection, or immunodepletion. However, the mechanisms governing this regeneration remain poorly understood. We detail such a mechanism, centered on interleukin-22 (IL-22) and triggered by the depletion of

CD4+CD8+ double-positive thymocytes. Administration of IL-22 enhances thymic recovery. These studies reveal mechanisms of endogenous thymic repair and offer innovative regenerative strategies for improving immune competence.[86]

A several exogenous factors have been found to be effective in thymic regeneration: thyme herb, zinc supplementation, prolactin, stem cell transplantation, or administration of dexamethasone.[87, 88] The infusion of genetically modified donor T-cells after hematopoietic stem cell transplantation (HSCT) can drive the recovery of thymic activity in adults, leading to immune reconstitution.[89]

There are two major pathways for T-cell reconstitution: thymus-dependent regeneration and thymus-independent homeostatic expansion.[90] The former recapitulates thymic ontogeny and generates T-cells from bone marrow (BM)-derived T-cell progenitors that undergo positive and negative selection in the thymus. Therefore, T-cells generated from this pathway usually have a diverse TCR repertoire, are capable of responding to a variety of foreign antigens, and tolerate self-antigens. In contrast, the thymus-independent pathway usually occurs by expansion of residual mature T cells in the periphery, thus producing T-cells with a limited TCR repertoire and the possible loss of self tolerance. Therefore, the thymus-dependent pathway is generally a preferred pathway for T-cell regeneration.

Using a murine bone marrow transplantation model, it is shown that thymic-independent T-cell regeneration occurs primarily via expansion of peripheral T-cells and is antigen (Ag) driven since significant expansion of CD4+ or CD8+ transgenic (Tg+)/TCR-bearing cells occurs only in the presence of Ag specific for the TCR. These findings have important implications for approached to enhance T cell regeneration in humans and provide evidence that vaccine strategies could skew the T-cell repertoire toward a specific antigenic target if administered to thymic-deficient hosts during immune reconstitution.[91]

T-cell development in the thymus is dependent on the thymic microenvironment, in which epithelial cells are the major components. Thymic epithelial cells (TECs) can be divided into cortical (cTEC) and medullary (mTEC) subpopulations. The former are thought to mediate positive selection and the latter are thought to control the negative selection process in which potentially autoreactive T-cells are deleted.[92]

The decline of thymic cTEC is a prominent feature of thymic involution. Because cTECs support early stages of T-cell development and hence determine the overall lymphopoietic capacity of the thymus, it is possible that the lack of sustained regenerative capacity of cTEC progenitor cells underlies the process of thymic involution. The impact of thymic atrophy is most profound in clinical conditions that cause a severe loss in peripheral T-cells with the ability to regenerate adequate numbers of naive CD4+ T-cells indirectly correlating with patient age. It is shown that androgen ablation results in the complete regeneration of the aged male mouse thymus, restoration of peripheral T-cell phenotype and function and enhanced thymus regeneration following bone marrow transplantation. Importantly, this technique is also applicable to humans, with analysis of elderly males undergoing sex steroid ablation therapy for prostatic carcinoma, demonstrating an increase in circulating T-cell numbers, particularly naive (TREC+) T-cells. Collectively these studies represent a fundamentally new approach to treating immunodeficiency states in humans.[93]

Transplantation of the thymic tissue under the kidney capsule is another approach to rejuvenate the thymus. The generation of embryonic stem cell (ESC)-derived thymic epithelial progenitors (TEP) has important applications at both basic and translational levels. Although some molecules have been implicated in early thymic organogenesis, molecules involved in the development of TEPs and TECs remain poorly defined mainly due to the lack of a suitable system for these studies. Also, any medical advance in regenerating thymus, must take the gender and sexual health in full consideration.

DiGeorge syndrome

Chromosome 22, the first human chromosome to be completely sequenced, is prone to genomic alterations. Copy-number variants (CNV) are common because of an enrichment of low-copy repeat sequences that precipitate a high frequency of nonallelic homologous misalignments and unequal recombination during meiosis.[94] Among these is one of the most common multiple anomaly syndromes in humans and the most common microdeletion syndrome, velocardiofacial syndrome (VCFS)[95], also known as Shprintzen syndrome, conotruncal anomaly face syndrome, Strong syndrome, congenital thymic aplasia/hypoplasia, 22q11.2 deletion syndrome, or DiGeorge.

DiGeorge syndrome is caused by the deletion of a small piece of chromosome 22 at the q11 region. It is a rare anomaly and happens in one birth among the 4000. The syndrome was described in 1968 by the pediatric endocrinologist Angelo DiGeorge.

Salient features summarized using the mnemonic CATCH-22, include: congenital heart disease (40%), especially conotruncal malformations (tetralogy of Fallot, interrupted aortic arch, ventricular septal defect, and persistent truncus arteriosus); abnormalities (50%), particularly velopharyngeal incompetence (VPI), submucosal cleft palate, and cleft palate; characteristic facial features (present in the majority of Caucasian individuals) including hypertelorism; learning difficulties (90%); hypocalcemia (50%)(due to hypoparathyroidism); digestive problems (30%); renal anomalies (37%); hearing loss (both conductive and sensorineural); laryngotracheoesophageal anomalies; growth hormone deficiency; thymic aplasia or hypoplasia and autoimmune disorders; seizures and psychiatric conditions; skeletal abnormalities.

The syndrome is diagnosed with the help of fluorescence in situ hybridization (FISH), BACs-on-Beads technology, Multiplex ligation-dependent probe amplification (MLPA) or Array-comparative genomic hybridization (array-CGH). FISH is done on a blood sample.

There is no treatment for DiGeorge. The key is in symptomatic approaches. In children it is important that the immune problems are identified early as special precautions are required regarding blood transfusion and immunizations. Thymus transplantation or prosthesis can be used to address absence of the thymus in the rare, "complete" DiGeorge syndrome. [96]

Myasthenia Gravis

When in 1974 the Greek shipping tycoon, Aristotle Onassis, was informed about his fatal diagnosis (Myasthenia Gravis) at his age of 68 years, he asked the doctor: *"Do the old men die from rejuvenating?"*

Myasthenia Ggravis (MG), Lambert-Eaton myasthenic syndrome (LEMS), or neuromyotonia, is an autoimmune disease, a neuromuscular transmission disorder, occurring with or without associated malignancy. In MG acetylcholine receptors at the neuromuscular junction are destroyed, inhibiting the excitatory effects of the neurotransmitter acetylcholine on nicotine receptors throughout neuromuscular junction. The cause is unknown.

In the thymus from MG patients, T(reg) cell numbers are normal while their suppressive function is severely defective, and this defect could not be explained by contaminating effector CD127(low) T cells. A transcriptomic analysis of T(reg) cell and conventional T cell (T(conv) ; CD4(+) CD25(-) cells) subsets pointed out an up regulation of Th17-related genes in MG cells. These data strongly suggest that T-cell functions are profoundly altered in the thymic pathological environment in patients with MG.[97]

B cell-activating factor (BAFF) is important in the development and maturation of B cells and their progeny-plasma blasts and plasma cells. There is increasing evidence that BAFF is involved in the pathogenesis of MG. While the exact role of BAFF in the pathogenesis of MG is not clear, BAFF and its receptors may provide potential targets for therapy in patients with MG.[98]

Although the disease onset is most often between the ages of 20 and 40 years, it can occur at any age. Women appear to have the disorder more often than men. About 12% of the infants born to women with MG have neonatal myasthenia caused by antibodies passively crossing the placenta; this condition usually resolves itself in several days to weeks as the antibody levels decline. Therefore, MG must be distinguished from congenital myasthenic syndromes that can present similar symptoms but offer no response to immunosuppressive treatments.[99]

Symptoms: Certain muscles such as those that control eye and eyelid movement, facial expression, chewing, talking, and swallowing are often, but not always, involved in the disorder. The muscles that control breathing and neck and limb movements may also be affected. Symptoms of MG include ptosis, diplopia, restless legs syndrome, and muscle fatigue after exercise with advanced myasthenia gravis can display pronounced muscular weakness and difficulty sustaining movement.[100] The disease can exist as a generalized disease or can be restricted to just the extraocular muscles as ocular myasthenia gravis. Note that the generalized form usually affects the ocular muscles as well, thus producing diplopia as one of the common symptoms of the disease.

The ability of a short-acting (< 5 minutes) cholinesterase inhibitor (edrophonium) to reverse the presenting symptoms confirms the diagnosis of myasthenia gravis -- patients should show an immediate, short-lived improvement. Other tests reveal acetylcholine-receptor antibodies in 90% of the patients with the generalized form of the disease and in 50% of the patients with the ocular form, despite the fact that the antibody levels do not correlate with the severity of the disease.

Over stimulation of the neuromuscular junction (nerve gases such as sarin, organophosphate insecticides) can produce the same symptoms, so it's critically important to exercise care in performing the diagnostic procedure using the administration of a cholinesterase inhibitor -- the addition of the cholinesterase inhibitor would exacerbate the condition of a nerve gas victim.

Screening: A syringe is loaded with 10 mg; 2 mg is given IV, and if no reaction occurs within 30 sec, the rest is injected. If the patient has myasthenia gravis, muscle function improves suddenly and briefly. The test can also differentiate between myasthenic and cholinergic crisis: Patients with myasthenic crisis improve, but those with cholinergic crisis worsen. Because dangerous cardiorespiratory depression can occur, facilities to maintain respiration and atropine (as an antidote) must be available during the test.

Left untreated, the disorder may be stable or progressive. With appropriate treatment, myasthenia gravis can usually be effectively managed with little impact on life expectancy. However, about 10% of the patients have life-threatening respiratory muscle involvement.

<u>Treatment:</u> Due to the common antibody-mediated pathophysiology, immunosuppression has an important role in the treatment of MG. Cholinesterase inhibitors are used to manage the the disease symptomatically. Corticosteroids and immunosuppressive drugs may be useful to disrupt the autoimmune response. *Thymectomy* is helpful in patients with the generalized form of the disease, with 80% going into remission or using lower cholinesterase-inhibitor doses.

Pyridostigmine is first-line treatment in generalized MG. Response seems to be better in patients with acetylcholine receptor (AChR) antibodies than in patients with antibodies against muscle-specific tyrosine kinase (MuSK). *Pyridostigmine* can be sufficient in mild MG, although most patients need additional immunosuppressive therapy. If so, *prednisolone* is efficient in the majority of the patients, with a relatively early onset of clinical effect. High drug dosage and treatment duration should be limited as much as possible because of serious corticosteroid-related side effects.

As long-term treatment is needed in most patients for sustainable remission, adding *non-steroid immunosuppressive* medication should be considered. Their therapeutic response is usually delayed and often takes a period of several months. In the meantime, corticosteroids are continued and doses are tapered down over a period of several months.

There are no trials comparing different immunosuppressive drugs. Choice is mainly based on the clinician's familiarity with certain drugs and their side effects, combined with patients' characteristics. Most commonly used is *azathioprine.* Alternatively, *tacrolimus, cyclosporine A, mycophenolate mofetil* or *rituximab* can be used. The use of *cyclophosphamide* is limited to refractory cases, due to serious side effects.

Plasma exchange and *intravenous immunoglobulin* induce rapid but temporary improvement, and are reserved for severe disease exacerbations because of high costs of treatment. It is recommended that computed tomography (CT) of the thorax is performed in every AChR-positive MG patient, and that patients are referred for thymectomy in case of thymoma. In patients without thymoma, thymectomy can be considered as well, especially in younger, AChR-positive patients with severe disease. However, definite proof of benefit is lacking and an international randomized trial to clarify this topic is currently ongoing.

When LEMS is suspected, malignancy, especially small cell lung carcinoma is considered. These patients need a continued screening up to two years. In paraneoplastic LEMS, cancer treatment usually results in clinical improvement of the myasthenic symptoms. *3,4-Diaminopyridine* is first-line symptomatic treatment in LEMS. It is usually well tolerated and effective. When immunosuppressive therapy is needed, the same considerations apply to LEMS as described for MG.

Peripheral nerve hyperexcitability in neuromyotonia can be treated with anticonvulsant drugs such as phenytoin, valproic acid or carbamazepine. When response in insufficient, start prednisolone in mild disease and consider the addition of *azathioprine*. *Plasma exchange* or *intravenous immunoglobulin* is indicated in severe neuromyotonia and in patients with neuromyotonia combined with central nervous system symptoms, a clinical picture known as Morvan's syndrome.[101]

<u>Treatment side effects:</u> Selecting the correct dosage of *cholinesterase inhibitor* can be difficult, requiring the expertise of a physician experienced at treating this disorder. Excessive dosage of *neostigmine* or *pyridostigmine* causes weakness that cannot be differentiated clinically from myasthenia. The disease may become refractory to the drug. Thus, if a patient who has been doing well deteriorates, the cause must be determined with the IV edrophonium test. If the patient improves, the maintenance dosage is inadequate. If the patient worsens, dosage is excessive or the disease is refractory.

Surgical rules and nuances

The first description of the thymic gland was by Italian anatomist *Giacomo da Capri* (1470-1550). The Swiss physician *Felix Platter* reported the first case of suffocation due to hypertrophy of the thymus gland in 1614. The first indication of an association between myasthenia and the thymus gland was in 1901, when the German neurologist *Hermann Oppenheim* reported a tumor found growing from the thymic remnant at necropsy in a patient with myasthenia.

The report by Hermann Oppenheim led the German thoracic surgeon *Ernst Sauerbruch* to perform a cervical thymectomy in 1911 on a 20-year-old woman with a radiologically enlarged thymus who had myasthenia. He reported that the myasthenia was markedly improved after the surgery, but resection of thymomas in patients with myasthenia at that time was accompanied by a high mortality rate.

In 1936, *Alfred Blalock* performed a trans-sternal total thymectomy during a remission period from severe myasthenia. By 1944, he had accumulated experience in 20 cases, firmly establishing the role of thymectomy in the treatment of these patients.[102]

Conditions or diseases of thymus requiring surgical treatment include:

- *Myasthenia Gravis.* Thymectomy is indicated when medical treatment fails, in younger patients with short duration of symptoms and in patients who have difficulty tolerating the side effects of the medications used to treat myasthenia gravis.
- *Thymic mass* (thymomas and thymic cysts). The aim of resection of the thymus is to completely remove the thymic mass.

Anesthesia: Total intra venous anesthesia (TIVA) may preclude the need for muscle relaxants. Opinions on the delayed awakening after administration of *sevoflurane* and *remifentanil* anesthesia in a myasthenic patient undergoing trans-sternal thymectomy are controversial. [103]

Anesthesia for thymectomy can be classified into: muscle relaxant or nonmuscle relaxant techniques. The nonmuscle relaxant technique includes insertion of a thoracic epidural catheter in an awake patient followed by induction of anesthesia using *propofol* and *fentanyl.* Tracheal intubation is facilitated with spraying the vocal cords with 3 ml of 4% *xylocaine* and maintenance of anesthesia is achieved with oxygen in air and 10–15 ml of 2% *propofol* as continuous IV infusion drip. The use of a nonmuscle relaxant anesthetic technique for trans-sternal thymectomy provides reasonable intra- and postoperative conditions. [104]

The most important preoperative factor predicting the need for postoperative mechanical ventilation is the severity of bulbar involvement, usually indicated by significant dysphagia and dysarthria associated with borderline respiratory dysfunction. [105]

<u>Pre-operative preparation</u> includes several diagnostic tests. Computed tomography is almost always obtained pre-operatively if a mediastinal mass is suspected and includes contrast enhancement to evaluate the involvement of the nearby vascular structures. MRI is routinely obtained in the large volume of thymectomies.

<u>Technique:</u> There are a number of surgical approaches to the removal of the thymus: trans-sternal (through the breast bone), trans-cervical (through a small neck incision), trans-thoracic (through one or both sides of the chest.) The trans-sternal approach is most commonand uses the same length-wise incision through the sternum used for most open-heart surgery. It is espoused by surgeons such as Alfred Jaretzki and is the most commonly performed procedure due to its relative simplicity.

The transcervical approach is a less invasive procedure that allows for removal of the entire thymus gland through a small neck incision.

<u>Surgical details:</u> The "standard" thymectomy uses a partial upper sternal-splitting incision in contrast to a transverse cervical incision or a complete sternotomy with cervical extension (Figure 16).

1) A short incision in the skin of the anterior chest wall in the

midline running from just below the sternal notch to the third interspace (at the level of the space between the 3rd and 4th ribs is made with a No. 10 blade).

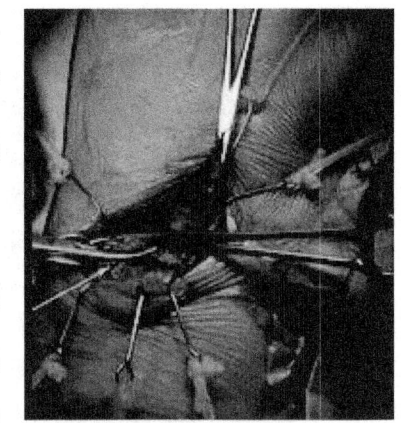

2) A sternal dissection is performed through the subcutaneous tissues with the Bovie cautery.

3) A sternal saw is used to divide the sternum to the third intercostal space and to completely to divide the manubrium.

Figure 16: Cervical incision with dissection of strap muscles.

4) A sternal retractor is placed, opened. The top of the incision is retracted toward the head (cephalad) Figure 17).

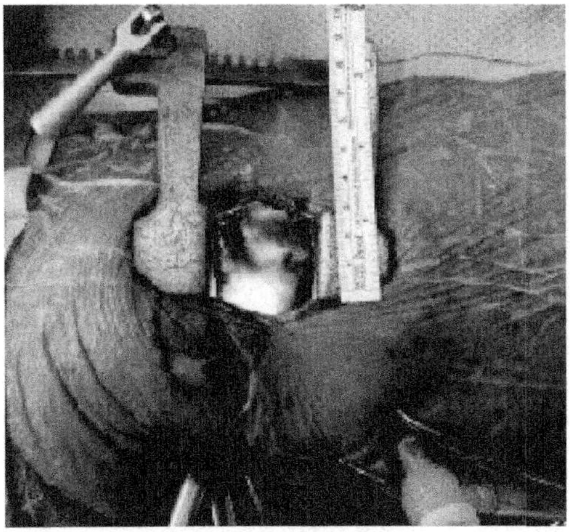

Figure 17: **The sternal retractor is placed; the top of the incisions is retracted cephalad.**

5) The anterior surface of the thymus is visualized and an inspection for a thymoma is undertaken (Figure 18).

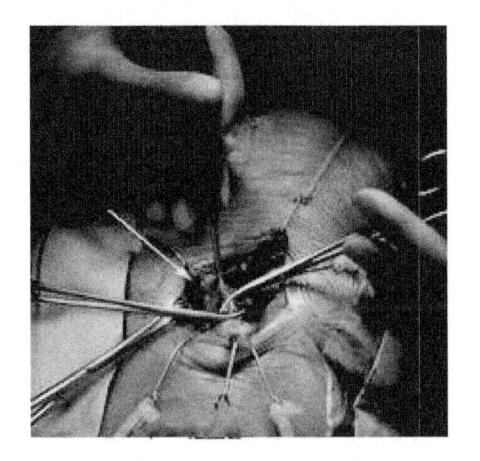

6) If a thymoma is found a complete sternotomy is required so

Figure 18: Superior pole of the thymus dissected into the mediastinum.

that a radical excision of the thymus can be performed.

7) Using both blunt and sharp dissection the edges of the thymus are freed from the pericardium (Figure 19).

8) Care must be taken when removing the thymus from the bilateral mediastinal pleura.

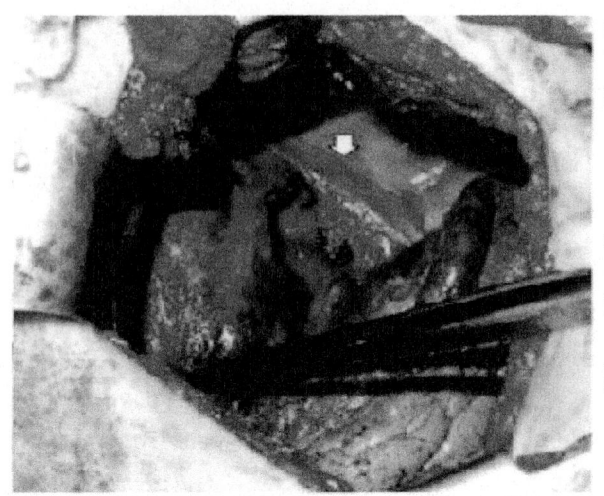

Figure 19: **The thymus freed from the pericardium**

9) Care must be taken to identified the phrenic nerves running on both sides of the surgical field and to avoid injuring these structures.

10) After mobilizing the thymus from the pericardium and pleural surfaces the lower poles should be easily retracted cephalad.

11) At the lateral margins of the thymus the internal mammary arteries are identified (Figure 20).

12) These are doubly ligated (tied) with 2-0 silk ties and divided.

13) The cervical extensions of each thymic lobe are removed with the body of the thymus by gentle traction and division of the thryothymic ligament.

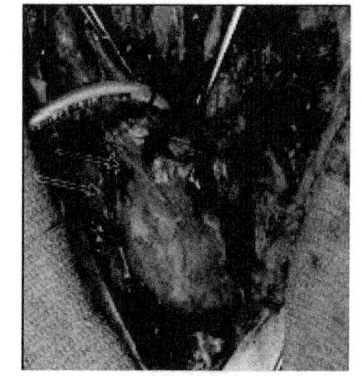

Figure 20: **Internal mammary arteries**

14) The thymic vein emptying into the innominate vein is visualized and doubly-ligated with silk ties.

15) The thymus is then removed.

16) If at any point of the dissection there is a thymic mass discovered (Figure 21) a full sternotomy is usually done.

17) If there is is adherence or invasion of the mass into an adjacent structure the thymus tissue is removed *en bloc* if possible.

18) Tissue specimens should be sent to the pathology lab for frozen section analysis to assure tumor-free margins if possible.

19) Before closing a thoracostomy drainage tube is placed in the anterior mediastinum.

20) The sternum is then reapproximated with sternal wires and the subcutaneous tissue is closed with a 2-0 Vicryl stitch and the skin is closed using a running 4-0 Monocryl subcuticular suture.

The Japanese practicioners offer a minimally invasive

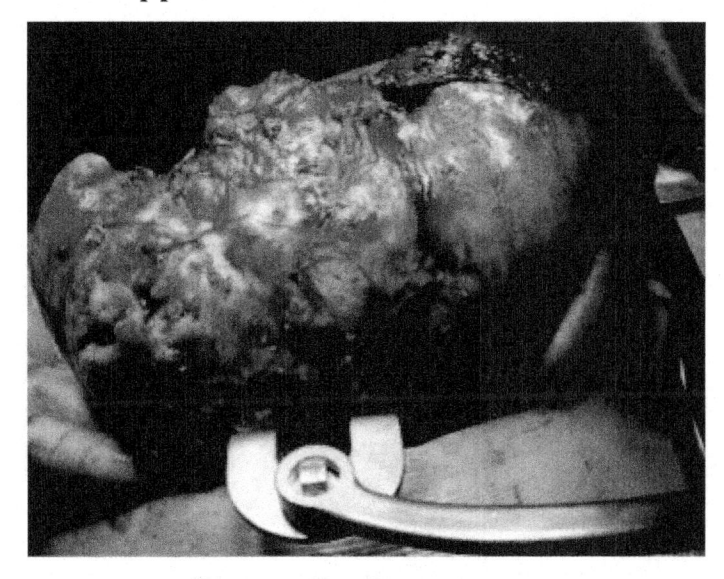

Figure 21: **Thymoma**

surgery using video-assisted thoracic surgery (VATS) for thymic diseases (Figure 22, 23).

This procedure has been modified from sternum-lifting thoracoscopic surgery with mini-thoracotomy to complete thoracoscopic surgery. Indications include benign thymic disease, non-invasive thymoma or myasthenia gravis (MG). Complications may include phrenic nerve palsy, and postoperative bleeding in the rare cases. The ultrasonic devices are always in use during the procedure. No recurrences have been identified in any cases. The VATS thymectomy appears acceptable as a less-invasive procedure with less pain and rapid recovery.[106] The same group of head and neck surgeons suggest a different non-invasive method of hymectomy, performed using intercostal and infrasternal approach with a sternum-elevator. Indications of this method tare benign thymic lesions (mature teratoma, thymic cyst and MG) and small thymoma (non-invasive Masaoka stage I-II, less than 5 cm in diameter and nontouching to the left brachiocephalic vein). New bipolar vessel sealing system

Figure 22: **VATS**

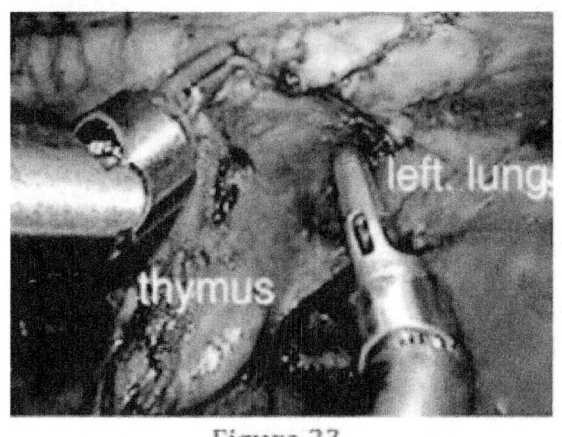

Figure 23

(LigaSure V) is safer and more useful than metal clip and ultrasonic coagulator in VATS for thymic vein sealing, extraction of upper poles of thymus and incision of mediastinal pleura near phrenic nerve.

Thymectomy benefits nearly 96% of patients: 46% develop complete remission, 50% are asymptomatic or improve on therapy, and 4% remain the same. The time from diagnosis to surgery is shorter than 8 months, and mild or moderate myasthenic symptoms are the main prognostic factors that predict the best outcome after thymectomy.

Surgeons conclude that the VATS thymectomy should be useful from the standpoint of less invasive, less pain, rapid recovery, and good cosmetic results.[107]

INDEX

Adaptive immunity		6, 7, 9, 55
Adventitia		13
Acetylcholine receptor	AChR	91, 92
Acquired immunodeficiency syndrome	AIDS	24
Adipocyte		7, 54
Anesthesia		95, 113
Anergy		8, 23
Array-comparative genomic hybridization	A-CGH	87
Ataxia telangiectasia		24
Autoimmune		12, 35, 53, 55, 72, 84-88, 91, 113
Autoimmune regulator gene	AIRE	14, 77
Azathioprine		92, 93
Basophils		20-22
B-cells		18-21, 37, 67, 70, 71, 89
B- cell activating factor	BAFF	89
Brachiocephalic vein	BV	14, 101
Bruton (X-linked)		21

agammaglobulinemia

3rd branchial pouch		14, 15
C1 esterase inhibitor deficiency		26
CD4+ T-cells		6, 8, 19, 22, 23, 48, 83, 85
CD8+ T-cells		6, 8, 17, 19, 22, 23, 71, 83
CD56+		17
CD40-CD40 ligand		21
Chakra		42, 46
Co-stimulatory signal	B7	23
Common Variable Immunodeficiency		21
Complement (C1, C2, C3, C3a, C3b, C4, C5a, C5b, C5b-9)		4, 11, 21, 25, 26
Cortex		7, 65
Corticomedullary junction		6, 7, 14, 65
Copy-number variants	CNV	86
Cyclosporine A	CA	92
Decay-accelerating factor (CD55) deficiency		26
Dendritic cells		4, 10, 17, 19, 55

DiGeorge syndrome		2, 86, 87
3,4-Diaminopyridine		93
Double-positive thymocyte	DPT	7, 8
Eosinophil		17, 24
Fluorescence in situ hybridization	FISH	87
FMS-like tyrosine kinase	FLT	8
Glucocorticoids	GCs	53, 63
Goodpasture disease		19
Hashimoto thyroiditis		19
Hassall corpuscle		11, 12, 49
Hematopoietic stem cell transplantation	HSCT	83
Hereditary angioedema		26
Human growth hormone	rHGH	49, 67, 87, 118
Hyper IgM syndrome		22
Hyperglycemia		38, 107
Hypoglossi nerve		14
Hypothalamic-pituitary-adrenal axis	HPA	51, 53, 63, 75
Immunocompetent		6
Innate immunity		46, 55
Insulin-like growth factor	IGF	68, 69

Interleukin (1-12)	IL	48, 75, 83, 106, 107
Lambert-Eaton myasthenic syndrome	LEMS	88, 92, 93
Leptin		54-56, 108
Leukemia inhibitory factor	LIF	51, 52
Lipopolysaccharide	LPS	63, 68
Macrophages		4, 16, 19, 23, 24, 37, 38, 49, 61, 70
Magnetic resonance imaging	MRI	48, 96
Major histocompatibility complex I	MHC-I	8, 18, 66
Major histocompatibility complex II	MHC-II	19, 21, 23
Mannan-binding lectin pathway		25
Mast cells		4, 17, 21
Medulla		12, 65
Monocytes		16
Multiplex ligation-dependent probe amplification	MLPA	87
Muscle-specific tyrosine kinase	MuSK	91
Myasthenia Gravis	MG	2, 88-95, 100, 101, 114
Mycophenolate mofetil		92

Natural killer cells	NK	55, 75, 110, 113
Oncostatin M	OSM	51
Opsonization		18, 20, 26
Paroxysmal nocturnal hemoglobinuria		26
Phrenic nerve		14
Pernicious anemia		19
Polycystic Ovary Syndrome	PCOS	76
Prednisolone		91, 931
Premature ovarian failure	POF	76
Progenitor Lin−CD44+c-kithiIL-7Rneg/lo		7, 8, 61, 85
Prolactin	PRL	68, 83, 109
Propofol		95, 113
Protectin (CD59) deficiency		26
Psychic attack		39, 40-42, 45
Pyridostigmine		91, 93
Recent thymic emigrants	RTE	8, 47-49
Recurrent spontaneous abortion	RSA	74
Relaxin		57-59, 109
Remifentanil		95

Rituximab		92
Selective IgA Deficiency		22
Severe combined immunodeficiency	SCID	25
Sevoflurane		95
Single-positive thymocyte	SPT	8
Steel factor		10
Sternum		9, 96, 97, 100, 101
Sternohyoidei muscle		12
Sternothyreoidei muscle		9, 12
Tacrolimus		92
T-cell receptor alpha	TCRα	47, 48, 84
TCR excision circle	sjTREC	48, 85
Terminal deoxynucleotidyl transferase	TdT	20
Thyme herb		16, 83
Thymectomy		48, 91, 92, 94, 95, 97, 100, 103
Thymic epithelial cells	TECs	68, 84, 85
Thymic involution		34, 37, 38, 50-53, 62, 64, 66, 67, 84, 85, 110
Thymic regeneration		38, 43, 67, 82-85, 112

Thymology		6, 30-33
Thymoma		92, 98, 100, 111
Thymopoiesis		7, 47
Total intra venous anesthesia	TIVA	95
Tumor growth factor	TGF	51
Urachus	VCFS	46
Velocardiofacial syndrome		86
Video-assisted thoracic surgery	VATS	100, 101
Zinc		78-81, 93, 111

REFERENCES:

1) Linkova NS, Khavinson VKh, Chalisova NI, et al (2011). *Peptidegic stimulation of differentiation of pineal immune cells.* Bulletin of Experimental Biology and Medicine; 152(1):124-7

2) Kuka M, Munitic I, Ashwell JD(2012). *Identification and characterization of polyclonal αβ-T cells with dendritic cell properties.* Nature communications; 3:1223

3) Haynes B F, Denning S M, Singer K H, Kurtzberg J (1989). *Ontogeny of T-cell precursors: a model for the initial stages of human T-cell development.* Immunology Today;10:87–91.

4) Haynes B F, Hale L P (1998). *The human thymus. A chimeric organ comprised of central and peripheral lymphoid components.* Immunology Research; 18:175–192

5) Kaye J (2000). Regulation of T cell development in the thymus. Immunology Research; 21:71–81

6) Lyman SD (1995). *Biology of FLT lygand and receptor.* International Journal of Hematology; 62(2):63-73

7) Lavini C, Moran CA, Morandi U (2008). *Thymus gland pathology: Clinical, diagnostic and therapeutic features.*

8) Miller JF (2004). *Events that led to the discovery of T-cell development and function-a personal recollection.* Tissue Antigens 63 (6): 509–17

9) Stahl-Biskup E, Saez F, Sáez F (2002). *The genus Thymus.* University of Hmaburg, Germany. Taylor & Francis (Hardcover)Huxley A (1992). *The New RHS Dictionary of Gardening.* MacMillan Press

10) Mises LH (2007). *Theory and history.* Yale University Press (Harcover)

11) Hülsmann GJ (2007). *Mises: The last knight of Liberalism.* von Mises Institute Alabama (Hardcover)

12) Tsuchiya M (1972). *Clinical prospect of Thymology.* The Keio Journal of Medicine; 21(3):127-45

13) Miller JF (1979). *Experimental thymology has come of age.* Thymus; 1(1-2):3-25

14) Sunwall MR (2005). *In the Praenumbra of Praxiology: Towards a Thymology of Tyranny based on the Psychology of Hegemonic Bonds.* Department of Anthropology, University of Hyogo, Akashi, Japan

15) Nishino M, Ashiku SK, Kocher ON et al (2006). *The thymus: a comprehensive review.* Radiographics; 26(2):335-48.

16) Furth van R, Schuit HR, Hijmans W(1965). *The immunological development of the human fetus.* JEM vol. 122 no. 6 1173-1188

17) Aw D, Palmer DB (2011). *The origin and implication of thymic involution.* Aging and Disease; 2(5):437-43

18) Johnson PL, Yates AJ, Goronzy JJ, Antia R (2012). *Peripheral selection rather than thymic involution explains sudden contraction in naive CD4 T-cell diversity with age.* Proceedings of the National Academy of Sciences of the United States of America; Epib Ahead of Print on Dec. 10, 2012

19) Singh J, Singh AK (1979). *Age-related changes in human thymus.* Clinical and Experimental Immunology; 37(3): 507–511

20) Barbu-Tudoran L, Gavriliuc OI, Paunescu V, Mic FA (2012). *Accumulation of tissue macrophages and depletion of resident macrophages in the diabetic thymus in response to hyperglycemia-induced thymocyte apoptosis.* Journal of Diabetes and its Complications; S1056-8727(12)00297-8

21) Aspinall R, Andrew D (2000). *Thymic involution in aging.* Journal of Clinical Immunology; 20(4):250-6

22) Aaronson M (1991). *Hypothesis: involution of the thymus with aging--programmed and beneficial.* Thymus; 18(1):7-13

23) Lynch HE, Goldberg GL, Chidgey A et al (2009). *Thymic involution and immune reconstitution.* Trends in Immunology; 30(7): 366-373

24) Taub DD, Long DL (2005). *Insights to thymic aging and regeneration.* Immunological Reviews; 205:72-93

25) Hudson LL, Markert LM, Devlin BH et al (2007). *Human T-cell reconstitution in DiGeorge syndrome and HIV-1 infection.* Seminars in Immunology; 19:297–309

26) Picker L J, Treer J R, Ferguson-Darnell B et al (1993). *Control of lymphocyte recirculation in man. I. Differential regulation of the peripheral lymph node homing receptor L-selectin on T cells during the virgin to memory cell transition.* Journal of Immunology;150:1105–1121.

27) Haynes B F, Hale L P, Weinhold K J et al (1999). *Analysis of the adult thymus in reconstitution of T lymphocytes in HIV-1 infection.* Journal of Clinical Investigations;103:921

28) Douek DC, Vescio RA, Betts MR et al (2000). *Assessment of thymic output in adults after haematopoietic stem-cell transplantation and prediction of T-cell reconstitution.* Lancet;355:1875–1881

29) Haines CJ, Giffon TD, Lul L-S et al (2009). *Human CD4$^+$ T cell recent thymic emigrants are identified by protein tyrosine kinase 7 and have reduced immune function.* JEM, 206 (2): 275-285

30) Izon DJ, Boyd RL (1990). *The cytoarchitecture of the human thymus detected by monoclonal antibodies.* Human Immunology; 27(1):16-32

31) Project Inform (2003). *The many faces of the human growth hormone.* The body pro: The HIV resource of health professionals.

32) Chandra RK (1979). *Nutritional deficiency and susceptibility to infection.* Bull World Health Organ;57:167–177

33) Chandra RK (1992). *Protein-energy malnutrition and immunological responses.* J Nutr.;122:597–600

34) Guo RF, Ward PA (2006). *C5a, a therapeutic target in sepsis.* Recent Patents Anti-Infect Drug Discovery;1:57–65

35) Sempowski GD, Hale LP, Sundy JS et al (2000). *Leukemia inhibitory factor, oncostatin M, IL-6, and stem cell factor mRNA expression in human thymus increases with age and is associated with thymic atrophy.* Journal of Immunology;164:2180–2187

36) Le PT, Kurtzberg J, Brandt SJ et al (1988). *Human thymic epithelial cells produce granulocyte and macrophage colony-stimulating factors.* Journal of Immunology;141:1211–1217

37) Le PT, Lazorick S, Whichard LP et al (1990). *Human thymic epithelial cells produce IL-6, granulocyte-monocyte-CSF, and leukemia inhibitory factor.* Journal of Immunology;145:3310–3315

38) Le PT, Tuck DT, Dinarello CA et al (1987). Human thymic epithelial cells produce interleukin; Journal of Immunology; 138:2520–2526

39) Betz UA, Muller W (1998). *Regulated expression of gp130 and IL-6 receptor α chain in T cell maturation and activation.* International Journal of Immunology;10:1175–1184

40) Wolf SS, Cohen A (1992). *Expression of cytokines and their receptors by human thymocytes and thymic stromal cells.* Immunology;77:362–368

41) Sano S, Takahama Y, Sugawara T et al (2001). Stat3 in thymic epithelial cells is essential for postnatal maintenance of thymic architecture and thymocyte survival. Immunity;15:261–273

42) Sobhani ME, Azad AK, Molla AW (2012). *A Review on Molecular Basis of the Role of Psychological Stress in the Development and Progression of Type 1 and Type 2 Diabetes Mellitus.* International Journal of Medicine and Medical Sciences; 2(5):117-122

43) Baumann H, Morella KK, White DW et al (1996). *The full-length leptin receptor has signaling capabilities of interleukin 6-type cytokine receptors.* Proc Natl Acad Sci USA; 93:8374–8378

44) Mandel MA, Mahmoud AA (1978). *Impairment of cell-mediated immunity in mutation diabetic mice (db/db).* Journal of Immunology;120:1375–1377.

45) Chandra RK (1980). *Cell-mediated immunity in genetically obese C57BL/6J ob/ob) mice.* Am J Clin Nutr;33:13–16

46) Lord GM, Matarese G, Howard JK (2002). *Leptin inhibits the anti-CD3-driven proliferation of peripheral blood T cells but enhances the production of proinflammatory cytokines.* J Leukoc Biol;72:330–338.

47) Matarese G, Leiter EH, La Cava A (2007). *Leptin in autoimmunity: many questions, some answers.* Tissue Antigens; 70:87–95

48) De Rosa V, Procaccini C, Cali G et al (2007). *A key role of leptin in the control of regulatory T cell proliferation. Immunity;* 26:241–255

49) Palmer G, Aurrand-Lions M, Contassot E et al (2006). *Indirect effects of leptin receptor deficiency on lymphocyte populations and immune response in db/db mice.* Journal of Immunology;177:2899–2907

50) Hick RW, Gruver AL, Ventevogel MS et al (2006). *Leptin selectively augments*

thymopoiesis in leptin deficiency and lipopolysaccharide-induced thymic atrophy. Journal of Immunology; 177:169–176

51) Gruver AL, Sempowski GD (2008). *Cytokines, leptin, and stress-induced thymic atrophy.* J Leukoc Biol; 84(4): 915–923

52) Howard JK, Lord GM, Matarese G et al (1999). *Leptin protects mice from starvation-induced lymphoid atrophy and increases thymic cellularity in ob/ob mice.* J Clin Invest; 104:1051–1059

53) Santora K, Rasa C, Visco D et al (2007). *Antiarthritic effects of relaxin, in combination with estrogen, in rat adjuvant-induced arthritis.* Journal of Parmacology and Experimental Therapeutics; 322(2): 887-893

54) Geenen V, Goxe B, Martens H et al (1995). *Cryptocrine signaling in the thymus network and T cell education to neuroendocrine self-antigens.* Journal of Molecular Medicine: 73(9):449-55

55) Seiki K, Sakabe K (1997). *Sex hormones and the thymus in relation to thymocyte proliferation and maturation.* Archives of Histology and Cytology; 60(1):29-38

56) Sakabe K, Seiki K, Kawaschima I et al (1994). *Effect of sex hormones of developmental of thymus tumor in spontaneous thymona BUF / Mna rats, with special reference to sex hormone receptors and thymulin (FTS).* Pathophysiology; 1(2): 117-125

57) Oner H, Ozan E (2002). *Effects of gonadal hormones on thymus gland after bilateral ovariectomy and orchidectomy in rats.* Archives of Andrology; 48 (2): 115-126

58) Bjelakovic G, Stojanovic I, Jevtovic-Stoimenov T, Bjelakovic B (2012). *Glucocorticoids, thymus function, and sex hormone in human body growing.* Nova Publishers, NY. Paperback.

59) Clarke AG, Kendall MD (1994). *The thymus in pregnancy: the interplay of neural, endocrine and immune influences.* Immunology Today; 15(11):545-51

60) Tibbetts TA, DeMayo F, Rich S et al (1999). *Progesterone receptors in the thymus are required for thymic involution during pregnancy and for normal fertility.* Proceedings of the National Academy of Science of the USA; 96(21): 12021–12026

61) Takashi I, Takeshi H (1962). *Studies of the influences of pregnancy and*

lactation on the thymus in the mouse. Zeitschrift für Zellforschung und Mikroskopische Anatomie; 57(5): 667-678

62) Napolitano LA, Schmidt D, Gotway MB et al (2008). *Growth hormone enhances thymic function in HIV-1-infected adults.* The Journal of Clinical Investigation; 118(3):1085-98

63) Gaufo GO, Diamond MC (1996). *Prolactin increases CD4/CD8 cell ratio in thymus-grafted congenitally athymic nude mice.* Proceedings of the National Academy of Science of the USA (PANS); 93(9): 4165–4169

64) Mello-Coelho VD, Savino W, Postel-Vinay MC, Dardenne M (1998). *Role of prolactin and growth hormone on thymus physiology.* Developmental Immunology; 6 (3-4): 317-323

65) Hasselbalch H, Jeppesen DL, Engelmann MDM et al (1996). *Decreased thymus size in formula-fed infants compared with breastfed infants.* Acta Paediatr;85:1029 –1032

66) Thompson JM, Becroft DM, Mitchell EA (2000). *Previous breastfeeding does not alter thymic size in infants dying of sudden infant death syndrome.* Acta Paediatrica;89:112 –114

67) Hasselbalch H, Engelmann MDM, Ersboll AK et al (1999). *Breast-feeding influences thymic size in late infancy.* European Journal of pediatrics; 158(12):964-7

68) Jackson KM, Nazar Am (2006). *Breastfeeding, the immune response, and nong-term health.* American Journal of Osteopath Assocication; 106(4):203-207

69) Carolis CD, Perricone C, Perricone R (2010). *NK cells, autoantibodies, and immunologic infertility: A complex interplay.* Clinical Reviews in Allergy & Immunology; 39(3):166-175

70) Allen EW (1911). *Experimental Station Report.* Vol. 25, Washington, DC

71) Ito A, Kano S, Hioki A et al (1986). *Reduced fecundity of Hymenolepis nana due to thymus-dependent immunological responses in mice.* International Journal for Parasitology; 16(1):81-5

72) Hiriart M, Romano MC (1986). *Human chorionic gonadotropin binding to rat testis receptors is inhibited by a thymus factor.* Life Sciences; 38 (9): 789-795

73) Gleicher N, Confino E, Friberg J (1987). *Is endometriosis an autoimmune*

disease? Obstetrics & Gynecology; 70(1):115–122

74) Bats AS, Barbarino PM, Bene MC et al (2008). *Local lymphocytic and epithelial activation in a case of autoimmune oophoritis.* Fertility and Sterility; 90(3) 849.e5–849.e8

75) Yan G, Schoenfeld D, Penney C et al (2000). *Identification of premature ovarian failure patients with underlying autoimmunity.* Journal of Women's Health and Gender-Based Medicine; 9 (3):275–287

76) Gleicher N, El-Roeiy A, Confino E, Friberg J (1989). *Reproductive failure because of autoantibodies: unexplained infertility and pregnancy wastage.* American Journal of Obstetrics and Gynecology; 160 (6): 1376–1380

77) Haller-Kikkatalo K, Salumets A, Uibo R (2012). *Review on autoimmune reactions in female infertility: Antibodies to follicle stimulating hormone.* Clinical and Developmental Immunology; Vol 2012, ID 762541

78) Jasti S, Warren BD, McGinnis LK et al (2012). *The autoimmune regulator prevents premature reproductive senescence in female mice.* Biology of Reproduction; 86(4):110

79) Bogoliubov VM, Karpukhin IV, Bobkova AS et al (1987). *Treatment of patients with chronic prostatitis complicated by infertility by microwave (460 MHz) action on the area of the thyroid and thymus glands.* Voprosy Kurortologii, fiziooterapii, i lechebnoi fizicheskoi kultury (in Russian) ; (3):15-8

80) Imade GE, Baker HW, Kretser DM, Hedger MP (1997). *Immunosuppressive activities in the seminal plasma of infertile men: relationship to sperm antibodies and autoimmunity.* Human Reproduction; 12(2):256-262

81) Mitchell WA, Meng I, Nicholson SA, Aspinall (2006). Thymic output, ageing and zinc. Biogerontology;7(5-6):461-70

82) Golden MH, Jackson A, Golden BE (1977). *Effect of zinc on thymus of recently malnourished children.* The Lancet; 310 (8047): 1057-159

83) Dardenne M, Boukaiba N, Gagnerault MC et al (1993). *Restoration of the thymus in aging mice by in vivo zinc supplementation.* Clinical Immunology and Immunopathology; 66(2):127-35

84) Dudakov JA, Hanash AM, Jenq RR et al (2012). *Interleukin-22 drives endogenous thymic regeneration in mice.* Science; 336 (6077):91-95

85) Boersma W, Betel I (1979). *Thymic regeneration after dexamethasone treatment as a model for subpopulation development.* European Journal of immunology; 9(1):45-52

86) Bhandoola A, Artis D (2012). *Immunology. Rebuilding the thymus.* Science; 336(6077):40-1

87) Vago L, Oliveira G, Bondanza A et al (2012). *T-cell suicide gene therapy prompts thymic renewal in adults after hematopoietic stem cell transplantation.* Blood; 120(9):1820-30

88) Williams KM, Hakim FT, Gress RE. (2007). *T-cell immune reconstitution following lymphodepletion.* Semin Immunol; 19:318-30.

89) Anderson G, Jenkinson WE, Jones T et al (2006). *Establishment and functioning of intrathymicmicroenvironments.* Immunology Review; 209:10-27

90) Mackall CL, Bare CV, Granger LA et al (1996). *Thymic-independent T-cell regeneration occurs via antigen-driven expansion of peripheral T-cells resulting in a repertoire that is limited in diversity and prone to skewing.* The Journal of Immunology; 156(12): 4609-4616

91) Sutherland JS Goldberg GL Hammett MV et al (2005). *Activation of thymic regeneration in mice and humans following androgen blockade.* The Journal of Immunology; 175(4): 2741-2753

92) Yu S, Graf WD, Shprintzen RJ (2012). *Genomic disorders on chromosome 22.* Current Opinion in Pediatrics; 24(6):665-71

93) Gul A, Gungorduk K, Turan I et al (2012). *Prenatal diagnosis of 22q11.2 deletion syndrome in twin pregnancy: A case report.* Journal of Clinical Ultrasound (JCU); Epub ahead of Print, Sept. 20

94) DiGeorge AM (1968). *Congenital absence of the thymus and its immunologic consequences: concurrence with congenital hypoparathyroidism.* IV(1). White Plains, NY: March of Dimes-Birth Defects Foundation:116-21

95) Gradolatto A, Nazzal D, Foti M et al (2012). *Defects of immunoregulatory mechanisms in myasthenia gravis: role of IL-17.* Annals of the New York Academy of Sciences; 1274(1):40-7

96) Lisak RP, Ragheb S (2012). *The role of B cell-activating factor in autoimmune myasthenia gravis.* Annals of the New York Academy of Sciences; 1274(1):60-

97) Spillane J, Higham E, Kullmann DM (2012). *Myasthenia Gravis.* BMJ; 21;345:e8497

98) Sethi NK (2012). *Restless legs syndrome in patients with Myasthenia Gravis.* European Neurology; 13;69(3):149

99) van Sonderen A, Wirtz PW, Verschuuren JJ, Titulaer MJ (2012). *Paraneoplastic syndromes of the neuromuscular junction: Therapeutic options in Myasthenia Gravis, Lambert-Eaton Myasthenic Syndrome, and Neuromyotonia.* Current Treatment Options in Neurology; Epub Ahead of Print, Dec.21

100) Kirschner PA (1987). *Alfred Blalock and thymectomy in myasthenia gravis.* Tha Annals of Thoracic Surgery; 43(3):348-9

101) Fanzsa JM (2006). *Total tntravenous anesthesia with propofol and remifentanil for video-assisted thoracoscopic thymectomy in patients with Myasthenia Gravis.* Anesthesia & Analgesia; 103(1): 256-257

102) EL-Dawlatly A (2011). *Anesthesia for thymectomy.* Saudi Journal of Anesthesia; 5(1):1

103) Baraka A (2001). *Anesthesia and critical care of thymectomy for myasthenia gravis.* Chest Surgery Clinics of North America; 11(2):337-61

104) Matsumoto K, Yamasaki N, Tsuchiya T et al (2012). *Minimally invasive surgery for thymic disease.* Kyobu Geka; 65(11):955-9

105) Matsumoto K, Kondo T (2006). *Indication and procedure of video-assisted thoracoscopic surgery to thymic disease.* Kyobu Geka; 59(8 Suppl):742-8.

Printed in Great Britain
by Amazon